Basic Concepts for Qualitative Research

Other titles of interest

Qualitative Research for Nurses
Immy Holloway and Stephanie Wheeler
0-632-03765-2

The Research Process in Nursing
Second Edition
Edited by Desmond F.S. Cormack
0-632-04019-X

Basic Concepts for Qualitative Research

Immy Holloway, PhD, MA, BEd

Reader, Institute of Health and Community Studies
Bournemouth University

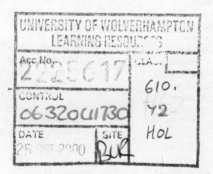

**Blackwell
Science**

© 1997 by
Blackwell Science Ltd
Editorial Offices:
Osney Mead, Oxford OX2 0EL
25 John Street, London WC1N 2BL
23 Ainslie Place, Edinburgh EH3 6AJ
350 Main Street, Malden
    MA 02148 5018, USA
54 University Street, Carlton
    Victoria 3053, Australia

Other Editorial Offices:

Blackwell Wissenschafts-Verlag GmbH
Kurfürstendamm 57
10707 Berlin, Germany

Blackwell Science KK
MG Kodenmacho Building
7–10 Kodenmacho Nihombashi
Chuo-ku, Tokoy 104, Japan

First published 1997

Set in 11/13 Garamond
by DP Photosetting, Aylesbury, Bucks
Printed and bound in Great Britain by
Hartnolls Ltd, Bodmin, Cornwall

The Blackwell Science logo is a
trade mark of Blackwell Science Ltd,
registered at the United Kingdom
Trade Marks Registry

DISTRIBUTORS
Marston Book Services Ltd
PO Box 269
Abingdon
Oxon OX14 4YN
(*Orders:* Tel: 01235 465500
        Fax: 01235 465555)

USA
Blackwell Science, Inc.
Commerce Place
350 Main Street
Malden, MA 02148 5018
(*Orders:* Tel: 800 759 6102
            617 388 8250
        Fax: 617 388 8255)

Canada
Copp Clark Professional
200 Adelaide Street West, 3rd Floor
Toronto, Ontario M5H 1W7
(*Orders:* Tel: 416 597 1616
            800 815 9417
        Fax: 416 597 1617)

Australia
Blackwell Science Pty Ltd
54 University Street
Carlton, Victoria 3053
(*Orders:* Tel: 03 9347 0300
        Fax: 03 9347 5001)

A catalogue record for this title
is available from the British Library

ISBN 0-632-04173-0

Library of Congress
Cataloging-in-Publication Data
is available

For my husband and children: Chris, Lynn and Britt

Contents

Acknowledgements

I would like to thank my editors Griselda Campbell and Sarah-Kate Powell for their continuous support and friendly advice. Jan Walker, Reader in Health Studies at King Alfred's College Winchester, and David Nicholls, Senior Lecturer in the School of Health and Community Studies at Sheffield Hallam University, reviewed the text, and I am very grateful for their constructive criticism. I particularly profited from my many discussions with Jan. I also owe a debt to Paul Atkinson and Janice Morse whose work stimulated my interest in qualitative research and has become a continuous source of ideas.

On a personal level thanks are due to: Stephanie Wheeler, my colleague, friend and co-author of *Qualitative Research for Nurses*, who shares her enthusiasm for qualitative research with me and who still finds time for debate and advice in her very full life; my colleagues, Mary Simms and Joan Revill, who read this book respectively for sociological content and language use; and Suzanne Hume, my Head of Department, who has always supported and encouraged me. Without my students I would never have written this book. It has been a privilege and joy to learn with them.

Introduction

Research has for long been an important task of academics, professionals and industry. With the increase of interest in a more customer- and client-centred approach, qualitative research has experienced unprecedented growth in the last two decades. Along with quantitative approaches, qualitative research is now used not only in social sciences such as sociology, anthropology and psychology but also in business and organisational studies. Professionals in the field of health, social care and education, too, see this type of inquiry as appropriate in their field because of its person-centred perspective.

It is in this context that the present text has been written. Denzin & Lincoln (1994: 1) state that 'a complex and interconnected family of terms, concepts and assumptions surround the term qualitative research'. I have attempted to explain some of these in an understandable form. I hope the book will be relevant for researchers who use qualitative approaches, in particular health professionals, educationists, teachers and social workers as well as students in these fields.

This text is more a handbook than a dictionary or glossary and can be used as a reference book. It consists of several parts. Initially there is an overview of qualitative research which is intended to be an explanation of methodological issues and to provide a lead-in as well as an overall context for the major part of the text. The next section contains the terms and concepts which are important for qualitative researchers. As well as discussing key concepts and terms I have also included sections on different approaches, and on research proposals and report writing. At the end of the book a list of texts can be found which should be helpful for those intending to carry out qualitative research.

There is, of course, a danger of 'trying to be all things to all people', but researchers can be selective in their use of the book. Although all approaches and concepts are not given equal space in my writing, I do not wish to imply that some are necessarily less important than others. My own particular interests have occasionally led me to extend certain explanations and to shorten others. This is due to my personal knowledge and background as sociologist. My greater familiarity with certain aspects of qualitative research has also influenced my writing.

The book has two aims:

(1)   It is meant to explain some of the key concepts and terms needed for understanding qualitative inquiry.
(2)   It should assist in writing research proposals and reports, and dissertations or theses.

The concepts and terms are arranged alphabetically for easy access. They include terms that are useful for qualitative researchers and also arguments to justify methodology, research design and research procedures.

Of course, my writing takes a strongly qualitative stance, but I believe that all approaches have their place. Qualitative research does not have priority over other forms of research, but it is a valuable way to gain access to the social reality of people.

Cross-references in the book are printed in *italics*. Important words or expressions are in **bold** letters.

Qualitative Research: an Overview

This overview attempts to trace the background of qualitative research and its development, and also some epistemological and methodological issues. It is meant to put into context the explanations of concepts and terms in the main section of the text.

Qualitative research

Qualitative research is a form of social inquiry that focuses on the way people interpret and make sense of their experiences and the world in which they live. A number of different approaches exist within the wider framework of this type of research, but most of these have the same aim: to understand the social reality of individuals, groups and cultures. Researchers use qualitative approaches to explore the behaviour, perspectives and experiences of the people they study. The basis of qualitative research lies in the interpretive approach to social reality.

The interpretive model

The interpretive or interpretivist model has its roots in philosophy and the human sciences, particularly in history and anthropology. The approach centres on the way in which human beings interpret and make sense of their subjective reality. Social scientists do not approach people as individual entities who exist in a vacuum. Instead they explore the worlds of people within the whole of their life context. Social scientists who focus on this model believe that understanding human experiences is as important as focusing on explanation, prediction and control. The interpretive model has a long history, from nineteenth century historians to Weberian sociology and George Herbert Mead's social psychology.

The interpretivist view can be linked to Weber's *Verstehen* approach. Philosophers such as Dilthey (1833–1911) considered that the social sciences need not imitate the natural sciences; they should instead emphasise empathetic understanding. Weber too, was well aware of the two approaches that existed in the nineteenth century (this was the time of the 'Methodenstreit' – the conflict between methods). The concept of 'Verstehen' – understanding something in its context – has elements of empathy, not in the psychological sense as intuitive and non-conscious feeling, but as reflective reconstruction and interpretation of the action of others. Weber believed that social scientists should be concerned with the interpretive understanding of human beings. He claimed that meaning can be found in the intentions and goals of the individual.

Weber argued that 'understanding' in the social sciences is inherently different from 'explanation' in the natural sciences, and he differentiated between the nomothetic, rule-governed methods of the latter and idiographic methods which are not linked to the general laws of nature but to the actions of human beings. Weber believed that numerically measured probability is quantitative only, and he wanted to stress that social science concerns itself with the qualitative. We should treat the people we study, he advised, 'as if they were human beings' and try to gain access to their experiences and perceptions by listening to them and observing them. Although Weber did not have a direct impact on early qualitative researchers, contrary to the beliefs of some social scientists (Platt, 1985), he did influence the sociologist Schütz and ethnomethodology, as well as later writers such as Denzin and Douglas, and his ideas have helped shape the qualitative perspective through them. Sociologists developed further the interpretive perspective that initially stemmed from the writings of Mead, Weber, Schütz and others in the early twentieth century.

Present-day interpretivists claim that the experiences of people are essentially context-bound: that is, they cannot be free from time and location or the mind of the human actor. Researchers must understand the socially constructed nature of the world and realise that values and interests become part of the research process. Complete objectivity and neutrality are impossible to achieve; the values of researchers and participants can become an integral part of the research (Smith, 1983). Researchers are not divorced from the phenomenon under study. This means reflexivity on their part; they must take into account their own position in the setting and situation as the researcher is the main research tool. Language itself is context-bound and depends on the researchers' and informants' values and social location. Detailed replication or duplication of a piece of research is impossible because the research relationship, history and location of participants differ in each study.

Qualitative methodology is not completely precise because human beings do not always act logically or predictably. Investigators in qualitative inquiry turn to the human participants for guidance, control and direction throughout the research. Rigour and order are, of course, important for the research to be scientific. However, the social world is not orderly or systematic; therefore it is all the more important that the researcher proceeds in a well structured and systematic way.

The historical background

Qualitative research has its roots in anthropology and sociology. As a method of inquiry, it was first used by anthropologists and sociologists in the early decades of the twentieth century, although it existed in a non-structured form much earlier; after all, researchers tried to find out about cultures and groups a long time before then, both in their own and foreign settings, and told stories of their experiences. In the 1920s and 1930s, however, social anthropologists such as Malinowski (1922) and Mead (1935), among others, and sociologists of the Chicago School, such as Park & Burgess (1925), adopted more focused approaches. At that time qualitative research was still relatively unsystematic and journalistic in style. Researchers reported from the 'field' – the natural settings they studied, be they foreign places or the slums and street corners of their own cities – by observing and talking to people about their lives.

Since the 1960s qualitative research has experienced a steady growth, starting with the emergence of approaches from a symbolic interactionist perspective (Becker *et al*, 1961) and the development of grounded theory (Glaser & Strauss, 1965, 1967, 1968). Filstead (1970) edited a major volume of readings on qualitative research. New publications in ethnography such as Spradley's work (1979, 1980) also gave impetus to this type of approach. Most of the research was carried out by sociologists and anthropologists, and academics and professionals in the education and health care fields adapted these approaches for their own areas. Earlier journalistic methods were abandoned because they were seen to lack rigour.

Much of the work originated in North America. The journal *Qualitative Sociology* was first published in 1978, and *International Journal for Qualitative Studies in Education* in 1988. In 1994, Denzin & Lincoln edited the comprehensive *Handbook of Qualitative Research*. In Britain, qualitative research became fashionable through its use in educational sociology in the 1970s and 1980s (Woods, 1979; Hammersley, 1983; Delamont, 1984; Burgess, 1985) and the text by Hammersley & Atkinson (1983) of which a second edition has now been published (1995). At that time health professionals, in particular, saw qualitative research as a type of inquiry appropriate and relevant to their work (Webb, 1984; Field & Morse, 1985; Leininger, 1985; Melia, 1987), and in the 1980s and 1990s this work has grown rapidly (for instance, Morse, 1991a, 1994; Smith, 1992; Benner, 1994). These are only a few of the many textbooks in education and nursing about qualitative research. In medicine, qualitative approaches are slowly becoming respectable but have not yet been wholly accepted as an alternative form of research. However, a book edited by Crabtree & Miller (1992) and a series of articles in the *British Medical Journal* by sociologists compiled in a small volume explained its use and made doctors more conscious of qualitative research (Mays & Pope, 1996). Significantly, the World Health Organization also published an overview of 'the concepts and methods used in qualitative research' (Hudelson, 1994).

Although psychologists had been relatively uninterested (with a few exceptions such as Harré & Secord (1972) and those in phenomenological psychology such as Giorgi *et al.* (1971) and Colaizzi (1978)), the attention of British psychologists turned to qualitative research when Nicolson (1991) prepared a report for the Scientific Affairs Board of the British Psychological Society (BPS) that urged a wider use of qualitative research (Richardson, 1996). The first, major, general text about qualitative research appeared in 1994 (Banister *et al.*, 1994). Books on specific approaches in psychological inquiry, such as discourse analysis, were published from the 1980s onwards (for instance, Potter & Wetherell (1987) and Potter (1996)). A special issue of the journal of the BPS was devoted to qualitative research (*The Psychologist*, Special Issue (8), 3). Smith *et al.* (1995) and Richardson (1996) edited texts which encompassed discussions of both theoretical and practical aspects of qualitative research. Qualitative approaches in psychology are now well established.

Researchers who take these approaches do not always use the term 'qualitative research'; they adopt different labels. Some call it naturalistic inquiry (Lincoln & Guba, 1985); field research (Burgess,1984; Delamont, 1992); case-study approaches (Stake, 1995); and interpretive – or sometimes interpretative – research. Others seem to use the term 'ethnography' as an overall name for much qualitative research (Hammersley & Atkinson, 1995). The latter highlight the lack of a 'hard and fast distinction between ethnography and other sorts of qualitative inquiry' (p. 2), and stress the diversity of qualitative approaches on the one hand and the epistemological and methodological similarities on the other. Although there are differences between qualitative approaches and strategies (Baker *et al.*, 1992; Stern, 1994), it is difficult to find clear distinctions between them. All qualitative research, however, focuses on the everyday life, interaction and language of people.

The methodology – the underlying rationale and framework of ideas and theories – determines approaches, methods and strategies to be adopted. Qualitative researchers choose a variety of approaches and procedures to achieve their aims. These include ethnography, grounded theory, phenomenology, conversation analysis, discourse analysis and co-operative inquiry among others. Some forms of social inquiry such as action research and feminist research often use qualitative methods and techniques.

The characteristics and aims of qualitative research

Different types of qualitative research have common characteristics and use similar procedures while differences in data collection and analysis do exist.

The following elements are part of most, though not all, qualitative approaches:

❑ Researchers focus on the everyday life of people in natural settings.
❑ The data have primacy; the theoretical framework is not predetermined but derives directly from the data.
❑ Qualitative research is context-bound. This means that the researchers have to be sensitive to the context of the research and immerse themselves in the setting and situation.
❑ Qualitative researchers focus on the *emic* perspective, the views of the people involved in the research and their perceptions, meanings and interpretations.
❑ Qualitative researchers describe in detail; they analyse and interpret; they use 'thick description'.
❑ The relationship between the researcher and the researched is close and based on a position of equality as human beings.
❑ Data collection and data analysis generally proceed together and interact.

The primacy of data

Researchers usually approach people with the aim of finding out about them; they go to the participants to collect the rich and in-depth data that may become the basis for theorising. The interaction between the researcher and the participants leads to the generation of concepts which are a product of the 'research act' (Denzin, 1989b). The data themselves generate new theoretical ideas, or they help modify already existing theories. It means that the research design cannot be strictly predefined before the start of the research. In other types of research, assumptions and theories lead to hypotheses which are tested and to the imposition of sampling frames whereas in qualitative research the data have priority. Although these approaches have their roots in a specific theoretical background – such as philosophy, symbolic interactionism, etc., the theoretical framework of the research project is not predetermined but based on the incoming data. The approach to social science is, initially at least, inductive. Researchers move from the specific to the general, from the data to theory. They do not impose ideas or follow assumptions but give analytic accounts of reality. They must be open minded though they cannot help having some thoughts about what they may find; Fetterman (1989: 11) claims that the researcher: 'enters the field with an open mind, not an empty head'.

While much qualitative research is concerned with the generation of theory (Glaser & Strauss, 1967), many researchers do not achieve this. New ideas may emerge from the data, but researchers cannot claim that they have produced or developed theory unless this assertion is documented. They usually do provide the interpretation of participants' experiences and gain insights into their world, describing 'the characteristics and structure of the phenomenon' (Tesch, 1991: 22) under study. Qualitative research is not static but developmental and dynamic in character; the focus is on *process* as well as outcomes.

Contextualisation

The context of participants' lives or work affects their behaviour, and therefore the researcher has to realise that the participants are grounded in their history and temporality. Researchers have to take into account the total context of people's lives. The conditions in which they gather the data, the locality, the time and history are all important. Events and actions are studied as they occur in everyday, 'real life' settings. Researchers must respect the context and culture in which the study takes place and try not to change it during their exploration (unless the aim of the inquiry includes change as an outcome, as in action research). If researchers understand the context, they can locate the actions and perceptions of individuals and grasp the meanings that they communicate to us. In a broader sense, the context includes the economic, political and cultural framework.

Immersion in the setting

Qualitative researchers use the strategies of observing, questioning and listening, immersing themselves in the 'real' world of the participants. This may generate descriptions of a culture (Hammersley & Atkinson, 1995). It helps to focus on process, that is, on the interactions between people and the way they construct, or change, rules and situations. Qualitative inquiry can trace progress and development over time, as perceived by the participants.

For the understanding of participants' interpretations, it is necessary to become familiar with their world. When professionals do research, they are often part of the setting they investigate and know it intimately. This might mean, however, that they are over-familiar and could miss important issues or considerations. To be able to examine the world of the participant, researchers must not take this world for granted but should question their own assumptions and act like strangers to the setting as naïve observers. They 'make the familiar strange' (Delamont & Atkinson (1995) called their book *Fighting Familiarity*!). Immersion might mean attending meetings with or about informants, becoming familiar with other, similar situations, reading documents or observing interaction in the setting. This can even start before the formal data collection phase, but it means that researchers immerse themselves in the culture they study.

Most qualitative research investigates patterns of interaction or seeks knowledge about a group or a culture. In clinical, social care or educational settings this may be interaction between professionals and clients or relatives, or interaction with colleagues. The research can be a macro- or micro-study: for instance it may take place in a hospital ward, a classroom, a residential home, a reception area or indeed the community. The culture does not just consist of the physical environment but also of particular ideologies, values and ways of thinking of its members. Researchers need sensitivity to interpret what they observe and hear. Human beings are influenced by their experiences; therefore qualitative methods encompass the exploration processes and changes over time in the culture or subculture under study.

The 'emic' perspective

Qualitative researchers explore the ideas and perceptions of the participants, 'the insiders' view', and search for commonalities. Anthropologists and linguists call this the emic perspective (Harris, 1976). It means that researchers attempt to examine the experiences, feelings and perceptions of the people they study, rather than imposing a framework of their own that might distort the ideas of the participants. They 'uncover' the meaning people give to their experiences and the way in which they interpret them, although meanings should not be reduced to purely subjective accounts of the participants as researchers search for patterns and commonalities. Qualitative research is based on the premise that individuals are best placed to describe situations and feelings in their own words. These meanings, however, are seldom clear or unambiguous (Addison, 1992), and they are not fixed; the social world is not frozen at a particular moment or in a particular situation but dynamic and changing. By observing people and listening to their accounts, researchers seek to understand the process by which participants make sense of their own behaviour and the rules that govern their actions. Taking into account their informants' intentions and motives, researchers gain access to their social reality. Of course, the reports individuals give are their own explanations of an event or action, but as the researcher wishes to find people's own definition of reality these reports are valid data. Although Dey (1993) warns us that we cannot always rely on accounts or on our own interpretations of them, we can often take our informants' words and actions as reflections of underlying meanings. The qualitative approach requires 'empathetic understanding', that is, the investigators must try to examine the situations, events and actions from the participants' – the social actors' – point of view and not impose their own perspective. This does not mean that the researchers never theorise or infer from observed behaviour or participants' words: they often do.

The researchers' and outsiders' view is the etic perspective (Harris, 1976). The meanings of participants are interpreted. There is 'elaboration and systematisation of the significance of an identified phenomenon' (Banister *et al.*, 1994: 3). The participants are part of the group or subculture in which they live, and therefore their words, actions and intentions can only be understood in that context. The individuals researching them have access to their world through experience and observation. This type of research is thought to empower the participants, because they do not merely react to the questions of the researchers but have a voice and guide the study. For this reason, the people under study are generally called participants or informants rather than subjects. It is necessary that the relationship between researcher and informant is one of trust; this close relationship and the researcher's in-depth knowledge of the informants' situation make deceit unlikely (though not impossible).

Thick description

Immersion in the setting will help the researcher use 'thick description' (Geertz, 1973). It involves detailed portrayals of the participants' experiences, going beyond a report of surface phenomena to their interpretations, uncovering feelings and the meanings of their actions. Thick description develops from the data and the context. The task involves describing the location and the people within it, giving visual pictures of setting, events and situations as well as verbatim narratives of individuals' accounts of their perceptions and ideas in context.

The description of the situation or discussion should be thorough; this means that writers describe everything in vivid detail. Indeed Denzin (1989a: 83) defines thick description as: 'deep, dense, detailed accounts of problematic experiences... It presents detail, context, emotion and the webs of social relationship that join persons to one another'. Thick description is not merely factual, but includes theoretical and analytic description. Strauss & Corbin (1994) go further by explaining that the emphasis in one of the approaches – grounded theory – is on conceptualisation rather than description. Analytic or conceptual description goes on to interpretation. Janesick (1994: 216) declared that description is the 'cornerstone of qualitative research'.

Thick description helps the reader of a research study to develop an active role in the research because the researchers share their knowledge with the reader of the study. Through clear description of the culture, the context and the process of the research, the reader can follow the pathway of the researcher and the two share the construction of reality coming to similar conclusions in the analysis of research (Erlandson et al., 1993). This shows readers of the story what they themselves would experience if they were in the same situation as the participants, and therefore thick description generates empathetic and experiential understanding.

Qualitative researchers are story tellers. Although the data collection and analysis are systematic and develop logically, as in all scientific research, writers present the findings and discussion in the form of a story with a distinct storyline.

The research relationship

In order to gain access to the true thoughts and feelings of the participants researchers adopt a non-judgemental stance towards the thoughts and words of the participants. This is particularly important in interviews. The listener becomes the learner in this situation, while the informant is the teacher who is also encouraged to be reflective. Rapport does not automatically imply an intimate relationship or deep friendship (Spradley, 1979), but it does lead to negotiation and sharing of ideas. It makes the research more interesting for the participants because they feel able to ask questions. Negotiation is not a once and for all event but a continuous process.

The researcher should answer questions about the nature of the project as honestly and openly as possible without creating bias in the study. The advice is to tell the truth without going into too much detail which informants might not understand or which may frighten them (Bogdewic, 1992). It is interesting that research books and articles differ in their advice on the relationship of researcher and informant. Some (for instance Patton, 1990) suggest a certain distance between the two, while others, such as Wilde (1992) feel that this could be a mistake because involvement and self-disclosure of the researcher facilitate disclosure and sharing of experiences from the participants. It is important for participants to realise that researchers, too, have human experiences just as they do and can empathise with them. The main goal of the meeting between researcher and informants is to gain knowledge.

The interaction of data collection and analysis

Another important feature of much qualitative research is the close connection between data collection and analysis. Without setting up a hypothesis before the study starts, the researchers collect the first data in the field and start to analyse them at the same time. They then develop tentative working propositions which they reformulate and modify in subsequent data collection. New concepts are developed throughout the process of data collection. They are continuously adapted and new questions formulated about the phenomenon as incoming data may challenge or modify findings. At each stage data collection and analysis interact.

The qualitative–quantitative debate: underlying philosophies

Social reality can be approached in different ways. Researchers will have to choose between a variety of research approaches. While they often make their choice on practical grounds, they must also understand the philosophical ideas on which it is based. The approach depends on the following:

❑ The nature and type of research problem
❑ The epistemological stance of the researcher
❑ The skills and training of the researcher
❑ The resources available for the research project

Researchers also have to think of the practicalities of the research such as their own skills and interests, the scope of the research and available funds and resources, all factors which may influence the undertaking of a project.

The initial choice is not easy. Approaches to social inquiry consist not only of the procedures of sampling, data collection and analysis. They are based too on particular ideas about the world and the nature of knowledge which sometimes reflect conflicting and competing views about social reality. Some of these interpretations of the social world are concerned with the very nature of existence (ontology). From this, basic assumptions about knowledge arise. Epistemology is the theory of knowledge. Minichiello *et al.* (1990: 102) state: 'Epistemological issues are concerned with knowing or deciding what sort of statements we will accept to justify what we believe to exist.' Methodology refers to the principles and ideas on which researchers base their procedures and strategies.

The following section will be a discussion about the epistemology of research approaches.

Epistemological concerns

Two main sets of assumptions underlie social research: they are referred to as the positivist and the interpretivist paradigms (Lincoln & Guba, 1985; Bryman, 1988). The use of the concept of 'paradigm' and the 'paradigm mentality' in qualitative research is, however, criticised by Atkinson (1995) and Delamont & Atkinson (1995).

Conflict and tension between different schools of social science have exi~ for a long time. In the positivist approach, the focus was on the metho~ natural science that became a model for early social sciences such as psyc~ and later sociology. Interpretivists stressed that human beings differ f~ material world and the distinction between humans and matter s~ mirrored in the methods of investigation. Qualitative research v~ towards the natural science model.

Positivism: the natural science model

From the nineteenth century onwards, the traditional and favoured approaches to social and behavioural research were quantitative. Quantitative research has its base in the positivist and early natural science paradigm that has influenced social science throughout the nineteenth and the first half of the twentieth centuries.

Positivism is an approach to science based on a belief in universal laws and insistence on objectivity and neutrality (Thompson, 1995). Positivists follow the natural science approach by testing theories and hypotheses. The methods of natural – in particular physical – science stem from the eighteenth and nineteenth centuries. Comte (1798–1857), the French philosopher who created the terms 'positivism' (and sociology), suggested that the emerging social sciences must proceed in the same way as natural science by adopting natural science research methods. One of the traits of this type of research is the quest for objectivity and distance between researcher and subject (*sic*) so that biases can be avoided. Investigators searched for patterns and regularities and believed that universal laws and rules or law-like generalities exist for human action. They thought that generalisations would be possible in all situations or cases (Hitchcock & Hughes, 1995) and made certain assumptions about human beings. Behaviour could be predicted, so they believed, on the basis of these laws. Even today many researchers think that at the heart of all research lie numerical measurement, statistical analysis and the search for cause and effect. They feel that detachment and objectivity are possible, and that numerical measurement results in objective knowledge. In this approach, the researchers control the theoretical framework, the sampling frames and the structure of the research.

Duffy (1985) declared that this type of research seeks causal relationships or links between events, although these links can never be proven. Popper (1959) claimed that falsifiability is the main criterion of science. The researcher formulates a hypothesis – an expected outcome – and tests it. Scientists refute or falsify hypotheses. When a deviant case is found, the hypothesis is falsified. Knowledge is always provisional because new incoming data may refute it. (There has been criticism of Popper's ideas but this debate cannot be developed here. It is discussed in philosophy of science texts.)

The approach develops from theory, and a hypothesis is often, though not always, established before the research begins. The model of science adopted is hypothetico-deductive; it moves from the general to the specific, and its main aim is to test theory. The danger of this approach is that researchers treat perceptions of the social world as objective and absolute, and neglect everyday subjective interpretations and the context of the research.

Nineteenth-century positivists believed that scientific knowledge can be proven and is discovered by rigorous methods of observation and experiments and derived through the senses. Chalmers (1982) asserts that this is a simplistic view of science. Even natural scientists – for instance biologists and physicists – do not, however, necessarily agree on what science is and adopt a variety of different scientific approaches. Social scientists too, use a number of approaches and differ in their understandings about the nature of science. Scientific knowledge is difficult to prove and is not merely derived from the senses. The search for objectivity may be futile for scientists. They can strive for it, but their own biases, experiences and often opinions intrude. Science, whether natural or social science, cannot be 'value free,' that is, it cannot be fully objective as the values and background of the researchers affect the research.

The critique of early positivist ideas

In the 1960s the traditional view of science was criticised for its aims and methods by both natural and social scientists. The new, and different, evolutionary stance taken within disciplines such as biology and psychology has gone beyond the simplistic positivist approach. One might call this a neo-positivist and post-positivist stance. Interpretivists go further. Lincoln & Guba (1990), for instance, argue that a 'paradigm shift' (in line with the ideas of Kuhn (1970)) occurred when earlier methods of natural science were questioned and new ways adopted: certain theoretical and philosophical presuppositions are replaced by another set of assumptions taking precedence over the model from the past. Natural scientists criticised the mechanical natural science view of the world, and some sociologists began to see it as socially constructed and defined.

Social researchers attacked the positivist stance for its emphasis on social reality as being 'out there,' separate from the individual. They maintained that an objective reality independent of the people under study is difficult to grasp. Quantitative research, in all its variations, is useful and valuable, but it is sometimes seen as limited by qualitative researchers because it may neglect the participants' perspectives within the context of their lives.

The controlled conditions in which traditional approaches take place sometimes limit practical applications. This type of research does not always or easily answer complex questions about the nature of the human condition. Researchers who use positivist or post-positivist approaches are not inherently concerned about human interaction or feelings, thoughts and perceptions of people but with facts, measurable behaviour, and cause and effect. These approaches are important and answer many types of research questions. Qualitative research is appropriate for different types of questions.

Conflicting or complementary perspectives?

Some social scientists believe that qualitative and quantitative approaches are merely different methods of research that should be used pragmatically according to the research question (Datta, 1994; Reichardt & Rallis, 1994). Others consider that they are incompatible and mutually exclusive on the basis of their different epistemologies (Leininger, 1985; Lincoln & Guba, 1985). Researchers sometimes use one or the other depending on their own epistemological stance. Bryman (1988) and Silverman (1993) address this dilemma by stating that neither school is superior to the other, and that an emphasis on the polarities does not result in useful debates. They do, however, stress that the approach depends on the intentions and goals of the researcher.

Many sociologists and psychologists still work in the positivist tradition. In much health, education and social work, however, the qualitative perspective is in ascendance. Some, like Atkinson (1995), do not believe that qualitative methodology represents a shift to a new paradigm. However, one might suggest that it is a coherent way of researching human thought, perception and behaviour (not new nor unilinear but more systematic and scientific than earlier ethnography or journalistic narrative).

Corner (1991) warns the researcher not to be simplistic about the assumptions of social science and overemphasise the differences between the methods which are based on these different philosophies. It must be remembered, however, that the positivist and the interpretive methods of social science have their roots in different assumptions about social reality. While early positivism is based on the belief that reality has existence outside and independent of individuals, interpretivists often claim that social reality, at least, is constructed and does not have independence from the people creating it.

Qualitative research as science and art

It is sometimes suggested that qualitative research is not scientific. Even as late as 1974 Easthope claimed that participant observation and life history are not scientific but artistic and intuitive, and that 'impressions' researchers gain through these approaches are not open to public scrutiny (Easthope, 1974: 88). He also asserts that 'science' does not deal with individual cases. Clarke (1995), however, comes to the conclusion that human relationships might be demeaned by involving scientific equations. She maintains that description of the social world cannot be truly 'scientific'. To be effective and cause change, this type of research should be creative.

This is not the view of most qualitative researchers who claim that qualitative approaches are scientific (for instance Minichiello *et al.*, (1990); Hitchcock & Hughes (1995)). Traditional nineteenth-century methods of physical science are not the only way to 'do science'. The question whether a particular research type is scientific or not is nevertheless problematic, and the answer cannot be given in an unambiguous, simplistic way. It is not just a question of 'objectivity'. Knowledge, even knowledge in the natural sciences, is located in temporality and culture.

It is claimed by neo-positivists that qualitative inquiry gives only a superficial picture of the world under study (unfortunately this is true for 'bad' qualitative research). Qualitative researchers refute this by stressing the depth of immersion in the study, and the length of the observations and interviews. Methodological rigour in qualitative research can be demonstrated through a detailed 'audit trail' where researchers describe the methods adopted and the problems encountered, giving a reflexive account. This way they open up their work to public scrutiny and critical examination. Rigour depends not only on the procedures but also on internal coherence and logic of the work. Validity, or trustworthiness, which demonstrates rigour is the extent to which the researcher's findings truly reflect the purpose of the study and represent reality. When the research is systematic and evidence-based, it cannot be described as merely impressionistic. In any case, there is no necessary contradiction between literary and scientific writing. Social science researchers agree that qualitative writing has some characteristics in common with novel writing and the arts. Shelton-Reed (1997) highlights storytelling as one of its most important characteristics, but this does not make the writers just entertainers. The writing is not 'merely' descriptive, it has explanatory power; it is interpretive; it is informative. Shelton-Reed claims that simple and narrative writing does not mean that the subject matter is also simple. Indeed it can be highly complex and theoretical. Communication of the content and context to the reader is as important as theory and methodology. One of the aims of the writer is to present the research as a coherent story. Atkinson (1992) rejects the criticism that ethnography resembles journalism. He claims that good and coherent stories in journalism or in ethnography are based 'on thorough research, ethically and conscientiously conducted, with a systematic review of sources and evidence...'. Hitchcock & Hughes (1995) maintain that qualitative research meets the criteria of science in its rigour and thorough analysis. This does not necessarily mean that the writing has to be difficult to understand.

Most qualitative researchers believe that qualitative approaches are scientific and open to peer examination and public scrutiny. Minichiello *et al.* (1990) argue that consistent and rational research cannot be labelled unscientific because it is based on a different world view from traditional forms of scientific inquiry. Systematic procedures, theorising and critical evaluation – all elements of scientific work – are involved in all good research. It is difficult, of course, to adopt a stance in which science is strictly differentiated from non-science. Science is shaped by both culture and history; research reflects the 'real world', and to be communicated it must be readable and understandable.

Key to Highlighted Terms

Italics	words in *italics* are cross-referenced and have their own entry in the list of terms and concepts
Bold	words in **bold** are important words or expressions
Bold italics	words in ***bold italics*** are important expressions which also have their own entry in the list of terms and concepts

Alphabetical List of Terms and Concepts

ABSTRACT

The abstract is a precise summary of the major points of a project and provides the reader with a brief overview of the *research question* and aim. It also includes a short statement of the *methods* adopted and the main findings of the study, giving information on the content. Researchers state clearly that they adopt a qualitative approach in their brief discussion of methods.

From the abstract, readers gain a clear picture of the aim, content, methods and main findings. As not everything is included in an abstract, writers should be selective about the content. In commercial or health service research for a funding body, the abstract is often called the **executive summary**. The abstract of a research project is presented in the past tense.

The abstract is written after completion of the study and appears on the page after the title but before the table of contents and the full report. Depending on the size and type of research, the abstract generally contains between 150 and 250 words. Usually it is no more than one sheet of A4 paper in single spacing. Writers should keep to the word limit specified. Abstracts of research articles or books are available on CD-ROM (compact disc read-only-memory) and other data bases. It is often the first piece of writing that readers see and is therefore very important.

Many funding bodies require an abstract for a research *proposal* which is shorter than the abstract of a report or thesis. This type of abstract states the goals and focus of the research and summarises methods that the researcher will adopt, and the potential use of the results of the inquiry.

ACCESS

Researchers must obtain permission for **entry** (or entrée) to the setting and **access** to the *participants*. Gaining access means that they can observe the situation, read the necessary documents and talk to potential participants. Formal permission is important in any research and protects both researchers and participants. Access to participants in qualitative research is a **continuing process** of ongoing inclusion and exclusion of informants and not a once-and-for-all procedure because the size of the sample is not always established from the beginning of a qualitative study but depends on the emerging concepts.

Access is sought in various ways. Some researchers pin up a notice on a public board in the organisation for which they work or put an advertisement in the local newspaper. Timmerman (1996) suggests that the place of advertising for research participants depends on the target population. She highlights the importance of making the advertisement or notice readable and interesting. The inclusion criteria must be clearly stated.

Some researchers ask permission from a group, talk to the members and ask them whether they wish to participate in the research. In the health professions this might be a group of people with diabetes or a carers' group. In teaching it could be a group of teachers of, for instance, languages; an example of participants in social work research might be a group of clients from a residential home.

The participants can also be approached through their immediate managers who explain the research and ask potential informants to participate. This strategy is not always advisable as participants might see the research as originating from management and be reluctant to disclose their thoughts.

Researchers have to take a number of steps:

(1)   They gain access to the setting
(2)   They make contact with people in the setting who can give permission for access and with those they wish to observe and interview, both *gatekeepers* and participants
(3)   They explain early and clearly the type of project and its scope and aims

The research might be prejudiced though, if all the issues are explained in great detail before the *interview*. This directs participants towards certain issues and they would not disclose their own ideas and perceptions. It can be avoided by giving them detailed information after the interviews. It is more difficult to negotiate access for observation because it involves the direct investigation of behaviour. *Informed consent* is still an important issue, and participants have to know details about the research. Sensitive areas for research, and vulnerable people such as mentally ill individuals, people with terminal illness or children, must be treated with thoughtfulness and care or excluded unless they are the specific group which the researcher intends to study. (See *ethics*.)

The researcher must be aware of the hierarchy in any system or organisation and know that conflicts between the interests of those at the top and those at the bottom of the hierarchy may exist. All individual participants involved should, of course, be asked for permission to undertake the study, and **voluntary participation** is essential. The researchers should realise that their presence and relationships with the participants may change the situation. This can *bias* the research and threaten some of the people in the setting under study. They can diminish the threat by getting to know the people in the setting and establishing a relationship of trust.

Researchers negotiate with the gatekeepers, the people who have the power to grant or withhold access. Gatekeepers are located at different places in the hierarchy of the organisation. Researchers should not ask just the person directly in charge but also others who hold power to start and stop the research. All gatekeepers have power and control of access, but those at the top of the hierarchy are most powerful and should be asked first because they can restrict access even if everybody else agrees. If they co-operate, the path of the research can be smoothed, and their recommendations might make others more willing to collaborate. However, researchers have to make sure that the participants do not see the research merely as a management tool unless it is a study commissioned by the people in a management position.

Gatekeepers deny access for a variety of reasons:

❏ The researcher is seen as unsuitable by gatekeepers
❏ It is feared that an observer might disturb the setting
❏ There is suspicion and fear of criticism
❏ Sensitive issues are being investigated
❏ Potential participants in the research may be embarrassed, fearful or too vulnerable

❏ Gatekeepers may not know about qualitative research and see it as 'unscientific'
❏ Economic issues – the research may take up too much time for the professionals involved

For these reasons researchers have to negotiate access with diplomacy and honesty, but they must also make the research *methodology* explicit and show that they follow a logical and systematic path.

ACCOUNT

An account is an explanation that individuals give about their behaviour. Through accounts they justify and, sometimes, excuse their social actions (Scott & Lyman, 1970). From participants' accounts, qualitative researchers are able to recognise cultural norms and rules. Social *actors* use this type of talk to make their behaviour and thoughts credible to themselves and others. Researchers gain information from accounts which are 'coherent constructions of the social world' (Coffey & Atkinson, 1996: 101). There are official and unofficial accounts. **Official accounts** are those obtained through historical documents written for public consumption, or sometimes through formal interviews when participants are fully aware of the answers they give and also take into account that these answers may be published. Researchers gain **unofficial accounts** through informal talk or after formal interviews when some individuals relate what they 'really' think.

ACTION RESEARCH

Action research is an approach in which researchers use intervention in a problem situation and then evaluate the impact of the intervention. If the results are unfavourable, the situation is changed. This type of research usually involves **collaboration** between researchers and practitioners. Action research is one of the most useful types of research. Carr & Kemmis (1986: 165) state its two major aims as being 'to improve and to involve'. Researchers and practitioners (or researcher–practitioners) attempt to understand and improve practice and its *context*. Therefore practitioners are generally involved in the design, the *data collection* and the *data analysis*. They also work to achieve the desired outcomes and evaluate practice.

Researchers who use this method believe in producing change in the situation they investigate. The common purposes of action researchers are: to change practice; to evaluate the change and to act upon it; and to develop and modify ideas. Action research generally involves small-scale intervention in a process or treatment in a work situation, and an evaluation of the impact of this process. Because of its small scale, the research is generally, though not always, qualitative. During action research, procedures and strategies are continuously assessed and renewed if they are ineffective.

Action research has its origin in the educational problem-solving approach of the 1940s in the USA; its first well known exponent was Kurt Lewin (1890–1947), the social psychologist. Lewin (1946) described a circular process for action research that includes planning, executing and fact-finding for evaluation. This research is meant to produce change in the setting under study. Action research has been used in industry, health care and education.

Without collaboration from the practitioners in the work place, changes in practice cannot be made. These changes are seen as necessary to solve problems in practice. Without development of theoretical ideas, the research stays arid.

Action research which involves researchers and practitioners on the basis of equality is called **participatory action research** (PAR) (Reason & Rowan, 1981; Reason, 1994). Planning action means setting objectives which researchers seek to achieve in collaboration with people in the setting. The traditional roles of researcher and practitioner are broken down; practitioners become co-researchers and full participants in the research process. Springer (1996) states the characteristics of action research as: **democratic**, because the participants themselves are involved and the research is collaborative; **equitable**, because participants are seen as of equal value; **liberating**, because this gives power to the participants, and **life enhancing**, because it helps people to express themselves. The practitioners collect information about their own problems, find strategies to solve them and convert the strategies into action. They then evaluate the changes they produced. There is a cycle of planning, taking action and evaluating. The original researcher – who is a facilitator – becomes a catalyst to enable the people in the setting to make an analysis of their situation and implement a plan for change. There are many examples of action research in nursing and business and in teaching. The analysis of qualitative action research is similar to that of other qualitative research, but in *cooperative inquiry* and participatory action research the participants are co-researchers. They plan, design, carry out and write up the research in collaboration with each other. Reason (1994) compares several types of action research which, though they are different, share some of the same principles.

ACTOR (or agent)

Social scientists see the social actor as a human being who actively creates the social world, not as a passive subject controlled by external forces. This term is often used in interpretive and qualitative approaches.

AIDE MEMOIRE

An aide mémoire (sometimes 'aide memoir' or check list) consists of key words or questions that remind the researcher of the areas of interest and the research focus. It is useful in unstructured interviews after researchers have asked the first broad question, and assists them in focusing on particular topic areas. An aide mémoire gives minimum structure to the interview and provides the researcher with guiding concepts so that the *dross rate* will not be too high while still permitting the *participants* to tell the story in their own way. Although the aide mémoire helps the researcher to focus on a topic area, it is not a rigid framework for the research.

Example of a question and an aide mémoire for health professionals

Main question
Tell me about your experience of hospitalisation

Aide mémoire
Feelings about the experience
Interaction with professionals
Perceptions of professional tasks
Visits of relatives, etc

ANALYTIC INDUCTION

Analytic induction is an approach to analysis that involves inductive processes (see *induction*). Analytic induction depends on a careful and detailed analysis of specific cases found through observation or interviewing (Manning, 1982); the *data* provide a basis for concept development and theory building. According to

Potter (1996), analytic induction consists of definition, tentative explanation, possible reformulation and generalisation. Initially a number of cases are examined and their essential features abstracted. At this stage *working hypotheses* are formulated, and the newly incoming data examined for fit. Researchers seek theories that can be applied universally, hence cases must be carefully examined so that negative or deviant cases can be accounted for in the emerging *theory*. Researchers build theory by constant construction and reconstruction. They change the theory until it can no longer be disconfirmed by new evidence and generalisations can be made.

Analytic induction was first used by Thomas & Znaniecki (1927) in their book *The Polish Peasant in Europe* and was developed by Lindesmith (1947). Analytic induction is not the same as the constant comparative analysis used in *grounded theory*. Glaser & Strauss (1967: 104) claim that those who use analytic induction attempt to establish universality but grounded theorists do not necessarily do this. Grounded theorists work with emerging categories whose main features are examined and wish to establish generality of theoretical constructs rather than the generalisability of the findings of the study.

ANTHROPOLOGY

Anthropology is the study of people within their *culture*. It is divided into different types: physical anthropology that has a biological base; cognitive and structural anthropology with its focus on cognition and language; and **social or cultural anthropology**. Social anthropology is the study of human beings in interaction. Qualitative researchers often work in the field of social anthropology. Anthropologists use *ethnography* as their method of research.

AUDIENCE

The audience for research is the people towards whom the research is directed. These are the researcher's peer group, for instance academics such as sociologists, psychologists, historians, etc. For those carrying out applied research, the target group may be practitioners such as midwives, doctors, teachers and social workers, or, sometimes, the general public.

AUDIT TRAIL (decision trail, methodological log)

The audit trail is the detailed record of the methods and decisions made by qualitative researchers before and during the research process. It includes a description of the setting, events and activities as well as a rationale for the research. The audit trail aims to provide the readers of the research with the information that will enable them to judge its trustworthiness and authenticity while carrying out an *inquiry audit*.

Related to qualitative research, the term was used by Halpern (1983) and developed by Lincoln & Guba (1985) and Schwandt & Halpern (1988). Sandelowski (1986, 1993) and Koch (1994) call it the **decision trail** because it traces the decision-making processes of the researcher.

The elements of the audit trail consist of:

❑ A description of the design with the aims and intentions of the research
❑ A record of the methods and procedures
❑ An explanation of the sampling processes
❑ A description of the data collection and analysis processes
❑ A record of decisions about ethical issues
❑ Excerpts from the data (such as sections of quotes from interviews or excerpts from fieldnotes)

Rodgers & Cowles (1993) advise that the context and setting should be described in detail. Through the quality of the audit process researchers can demonstrate the quality, credibility and rigour of their work. (See *inquiry audit*.)

AUTO-ETHNOGRAPHY

An auto-ethnography is the study of one's own culture. Many ethnographies in nursing and teaching are auto-ethnographies. For instance, teachers or nurses who study their own *culture* and write about it produce an auto-ethnography. The term was first used by Hayano (1979).

B

BASIC SOCIAL PROCESS (BSP)

The BSP is a social process which occurs over time. It explains changes in the behaviour of participants and presents the stages through which they proceed in their particular situation. It can be found through prolonged immersion of the researcher in the setting. This term was developed in the work of Glaser & Strauss (1967) and Glaser (1978) for *grounded theory*. The process has stages and demonstrates development over time; it is a type of core category. An example would be 'becoming professional'. Glaser refers to basic social psychological processes (for instance 'becoming') and to basic social structural processes (such as bureaucratisation).

BIAS

Bias exists when research becomes distorted for a variety of reasons. Qualitative researchers do not often use the term bias as they try to make explicit their own assumptions and predisposition from the beginning of the research. Indeed some feel that 'bias' is a **misnomer**.

Distortions may emerge for different reasons. **Researcher biases** are prejudices of researchers of which they are not always aware. Researchers are affected by their culture, education, group membership, gender, personal disposition or other personal and environmental factors, such as age and personality traits. They do not always recognise personal preferences and might spend more time with one person or in one place than another; they may also be unconsciously influenced by élite groups or particularly vulnerable participants. Value judgements that the researcher makes while writing *fieldnotes* could also introduce distortion. Researchers try to counteract bias by *reflexivity* and self-criticism and by converting *subjectivity* into a resource for the study. This is important because the researcher is the main instrument in qualitative research.

Bias in subject matter (Atkinson, 1990) occasionally exists in ethnographic and sociological research, because the study often focuses on the different and deviant. The choice of topic, the particular time in which the research takes place and the location of the research may also produce bias. For instance, social workers who explore the culture of drug takers may feel a strong reaction against these participants. They should not show their own prejudices because the participants are affected by these and might not tell the truth. For instance, a doctor who has a strong objection to abortion on religious grounds would not be advised to study this topic area.

Sampling **bias** may occur in the selection of the sample because researchers have adopted a particular stance or choose people who support their assumptions or preconceptions. Bias can also occur in the selection and interpretation of *data*; only those data might be chosen which fit into the overall framework of the researcher. For instance, if health professionals feel strongly against mixed-sex wards, the research report could be skewed if some data are left out. For example, midwives who have interviewed a number of women about the birth process cannot just select a sample of women who agree with their ideas about this. Researchers might not report the cases that do not support their ideas; this is sometimes done unconsciously, but if done deliberately it would be both unethical and 'bad' research.

Key informant bias can be a problem. Because researchers select only a small sample of *key informants*, the view of these participants may be untypical and not representative of the cultural members' ideas. Participants occasionally try to impress the researcher by exaggerating their information. For this reason, *saturation* in sampling can be important. Saturation means that sampling proceeds until no new data are generated (Glaser & Strauss, 1967).

Qualitative researchers do not find it difficult to avoid **contextual bias** related to interviews (Hudelson, 1994). They do not depend on specific areas in which they collect information, but they have access to the culture of the informant and immerse themselves in the setting. They do not have a fleeting relationship with the participants in the study but close links and can often recognise sources of bias.

Bias is different from error. The latter is the outcome of mistakes made by the researcher or participants.

BRACKETING

Bracketing means suspension of the researcher's preconceived ideas and previous knowledge about a phenomenon so that this can be examined without too many prior assumptions. For bracketing to take place, the researcher has first to identify these assumptions and beliefs. The mathematical term 'bracketing' was used by Husserl (1931) in his study of *phenomenology*. Researchers may make assumptions about their knowledge of a condition or a culture. They bracket their knowledge and assumptions so that they can enter the situation without prejudice.

C

CAQDAS (Computer-Assisted Qualitative Data Analysis Software)

The term CAQDAS was first used at a conference in 1989 (Mangabeira, 1996; Fielding & Lee, 1991). CAQDAS programs are specially built programs created by qualitative researchers, sometimes with the help of computer experts, to replace mechanical manual tasks of cutting, pasting and other processes in the analysis of data.

A CAQDAS networking project that is funded by the Economic and Social Research Council (*ESRC*) in Britain aims to provide information about computer analysis in qualitative social science research. It is directed by Nigel Fielding from the University of Surrey and Ray Lee from Royal Holloway College, University of London. The CAQDAS World Wide Web page allows researchers to access demonstrations of data analysis packages, information about training courses and a variety of resources. Seminars and workshops about computer-assisted analysis of qualitative data take place in the University of Surrey and Royal Holloway College (Lewins, 1996). (Specific programs, such as NUDIST, Ethnograph or Hypersoft, are not discussed here. They can be found in the relevant texts on qualitative computer analysis.)

CARD SORTING

Card sorting, a term used by the ethnographer Spradley (1979), means that researchers present informants with sets of cards on which participants list a number of terms or concepts. Ethnographers then can ask questions about these. This stimulates the informants to think about the word and relate other terms to it that belong to the same *domain*. It helps in the development of the organisation of data and analytical categories. Card sorting prevents researchers from imposing their own ideas. Through this they obtain more detail from the *participants* and examine the ways in which the participants' knowledge and thoughts are organised. Spradley (1979: 131) claims: 'Ethnography is more than finding out what people know; it also involves discovering how people have organised that knowledge.'

CASE STUDY

A case study in research is an entity which is studied as a single unit and has clear boundaries; it is an investigation of an organisation, an event, a process or a programme (Merriam, 1988). The term has changed its meaning over time (Platt, 1983). The term 'case study' is used for a variety of research approaches (Yin, 1993), both qualitative and quantitative, but in this book it describes the qualitative study. Much qualitative inquiry is seen as case study research, but case studies differ from other qualitative approaches because of their specific focus and the examination of individual cases. The boundaries of the case are clarified in terms of the questions asked, the data sources used and the setting and person(s) involved. The case study features in a number of disciplines, such as anthropology, sociology or geography, although not all projects on limited cases are case studies.

Case study research has been most popular in business studies, but is also used in social work and nursing. The case study in research is different from the one used as a teaching tool in business or health studies where a case is given to students for analysis and solutions.

Features and purpose of case study research

Generally, although not always, researchers are familiar with the case they examine and its context prior to the research. They investigate it because they need the knowledge about the particular case.

As in other qualitative approaches, case study research is a way of exploring the phenomenon in its context. Researchers use a number of sources in their data collection, for instance observation, documents and interviews, so that the case can be illuminated from all sides. *Observation* and documentary research are the most common strategies used in case study research. There is no specific method for data collection or analysis; the researcher can apply ethnographic, phenomenological approaches or grounded theory. The analysis of qualitative case studies involves the same techniques as that of other qualitative methods: the researcher categorises, develops typologies and themes and generates theoretical ideas. (See *induction*.)

Studies focus on individuals or groups with common experiences or characteristics. *Life histories* of individuals could also be interesting examples of cases.

Case study research can be an exploratory device. For instance, it may be a *pilot study* for a larger project or for more quantitative research. Cases could also illustrate the specific elements of a research project. Usually the case study stands on its own and involves intensive observation. The description of relevant cases can make a project more lively and interesting.

Case study research is used mainly to investigate cases which are tied to a specific situation and locality, and hence this type of inquiry is even less readily generalisable than other qualitative research (but see *generalisability*). Therefore researchers often study 'typical' and multiple cases (Stake, 1995). The atypical case may, however, sometimes be interesting because its very difference might illustrate the typical case. It is important that the researcher does not make unwarranted assertions about generalisability on the basis of a single case.

CATEGORY

A category in qualitative research is a conceptual label given to higher-order concepts which are grouped together. After *coding* the data, researchers put together clusters of similar codes and give them a label. Such a category might be 'searching for information' or 'interaction rituals'. The whole cluster of ideas about these areas has been reduced to a category. A **member-identified category** is the category with which informants in research identify themselves. For example, a student might use the term 'thrown in at the deep end' which expresses ideas about lack of formal socialisation into an occupation and frustration with the haphazard process in which it might have happened. **Observer-identified categories** are those which the researcher identifies and formulates. (See *coding*.)

CAUSALITY

A causal relationship exists when particular processes or events lead to specific outcomes. For instance, a causal relationship has been established when there is evidence that a particular type of upbringing leads to crime. Qualitative researchers believed in the past that their approaches did not examine causality. This has changed: some qualitative research does attempt to identify causal relationships. However, much qualitative research focuses on explanations which are not necessarily causal. Research often does, however, develop explanations for existing causal relationships, such as the one between health and social class.

CHICAGO SCHOOL

The Chicago School of Sociology was based at Chicago University, and flourished between the two World Wars. Its most prominent member was Robert Park who started as a journalist. It is known for its early qualitative approach to research in urban settings. Sociologists transferred anthropological research methods to their own *culture* and society. Initially, the Chicagoans, who were interested in social interaction, relied often on a single case, such as a group, a community or subculture (for instance a gang) with an emphasis on life in the city. This early qualitative research consisted of working 'in the field', the slums, bars and street corners of the city, observing people and interviewing them. Their main interest seems to have focused on these problems rather than on method. Researchers participated in the culture and believed in 'getting their hands dirty'. From an early journalistic approach, this research became more systematic over time. Much well-known work in urban studies originated in the Chicago School (Park & Burgess, 1925; Thomas & Znaniecki, 1927). This tradition was followed by such eminent sociologists as Whyte (1943) and Becker *et al.* (1961).

CODING

Coding in *qualitative research* means identifying and labelling concepts and phrases in interview transcripts and fieldnotes. The identifying label for the data unit is called a code. Coding is an early step in the analysis of data.

Researchers group closely linked concepts into *categories*. These are often more abstract than the initial concepts. After this stage, researchers collapse categories into *themes* or *constructs*. Categories and concepts are instances of these themes. (See also *grounded theory* for open coding, axial coding and selective coding.)

CONCEPT

A concept is a descriptive or explanatory idea, the meaning embedded in a term. A *theory* is built from a number of interconnecting concepts. (See also *sensitising concept*. This term is used by Blumer (1954), as a means of creating awareness in the researcher.)

CONCEPT MAPPING

Concept mapping is described by Maxwell (1996) as drawing a picture about the area of study that the researcher wishes to carry out. It is intended to be a tool for the production of theoretical ideas and the development of concepts and relationships between them. The concept map can be hand-drawn on paper or developed on a computer. Concept maps are continuously re-drawn as new concepts emerge. Novak & Gowin (1984) initially developed the term concept mapping.

CONCEPTUAL DENSITY

Conceptual density in qualitative research exists when concepts and relationships have been well developed and the emphasis is on conceptualisation (Strauss & Corbin, 1994). The concepts and their relationships are directly based on the data.

CONSTANT COMPARISON

The constant comparative method consists of a series of iterative steps in which the researcher continuously compares sections of data, incidents or cases. *Grounded theory* uses this type of analysis. In their original book, Glaser & Strauss (1967) explain that all types of qualitative information, such as *inter-*

views, documents and *observations* as well as the literature, are compared. They describe this process in four stages:

(1)   Researchers compare the incidents which are applicable to each *category*. While *coding* they compare ideas which develop within a category with those that previously arose in the same category.

(2)   Researchers integrate categories and their properties. From comparing incidents with other incidents, they go on to compare incidents with the properties of a category.

(3)   Researchers provide an outline for the *theory*. While comparing and linking categories they find patterns in the categories which help in the formulation of theory.

(4)   Researchers develop the theory. Researchers collate the theoretical notes which they have on a category, summarise them and develop major themes. Through this the theory is developed. (See *memoing*.)

CONSTRUCT

A construct in qualitative research is an abstract and general concept built up from specific instances or observations. A number of constructs assist in building theories. (See *coding* and *category*.)

CONTENT ANALYSIS

Content analysis is a form of analysis which is applied to the content of documents or other forms of communication. Holsti (1969: 5) cites a number of researchers who maintain that content analysis is always quantitative as it measures frequency, but he stresses that frequency is not the only valid criterion. The term 'content analysis' has broadened in recent years, and the idea is less restrictive than it was in the early days of its use when Berelson (1952) wrote about it. Qualitative researchers sometimes use latent and/or inductive content analysis for their data.

Manifest content analysis is a type of analysis in which researchers search the content of an interview or document for particular *concepts* and *categories* apparent in the data. The criteria for their selection and the coding system are established prior to the analysis (Krippendorf, 1980). Researchers count the **frequency** of words or concepts and/or the numbers of instances of action or interaction. The frequency determines the significance of a concept. Although this type of analysis is quantitative, it does have qualitative elements. Tesch (1990: 25) maintains that 'its conclusions are not statistical, they are substantive'. As an identified method of analysis, content analysis was first used by Berelson and Lazarsfeld, two American sociologists, although the approach has existed for a long time in a simple form. This type of analysis is not qualitative.

Latent content analysis is a search for meanings in the data which are not immediately obvious from listening and reading. The analysis goes beyond surface themes and appearances to underlying phenomena and their interpretations. Researchers demonstrate the inferred meanings of the interview or document data by giving excerpts from the data. The imposition of categories by the researcher before the start of the research prevents this type of analysis from being truly qualitative, although qualitative analysis has occasionally been called latent content analysis in the past (see, for instance, Field & Morse (1985)).

Inductive content analysis is a type of analysis in which researchers derive themes and constructs from the data without imposing a prior framework and without counting. While immersed in the data, they search for general patterns and generate working hypotheses (see *hypothesis*).

It is not easy to distinguish between different forms of content analysis. The term was used in the early days of qualitative research when particular approaches such as *grounded theory* or phenomenological approaches to analysis had not yet been fully developed. Although qualitative researchers use interview texts and *fieldnotes* from observation as data sources, it is probably better not to use the term content analysis when carrying out qualitative research as the notion might imply that frequency counts have been carried out.

CONTEXT

Context refers to the environment and the conditions in which the research occurs, and includes the social and cultural system of the participants. Qualitative researchers must have awareness and knowledge of the context, that is, have **context sensitivity** and **context intelligence**. The context of the data in qualitative research is essential for its interpretation as it has an impact on the research participants as well as on the researchers themselves. For instance, when researchers examine the interaction between health professionals and patients, they take into account the group membership and gender of participants because it affects the interaction. Another example: a woman's narrative about having a child outside marriage in 1945 might differ completely from that of a much younger mother who conceived a child outside marriage in the 1990s because ideas about the appropriateness of having children outside a marital relationship have changed. Documents such as letters or diaries can only be examined in their historical and temporal context.

Silverman (1993) uses the term contextual sensitivity. Through being sensitive, researchers recognise that institutions and concepts have meanings which differ according to context. He cites the institution of the 'family' as one example; the concept of family in the last century differs from the idea of the modern family. Silverman also stresses the active production of context by human agents. Researchers should be aware of this rather than making assumptions on the basis of their own situation.

CONTEXTUALISATION

Contextualisation takes place when researchers attempt to understand the *data* in *context*. Events and actions are seen as linked to each other and related to the context in which they occur. (See *context* and *decontextualisation*.)

CONVERSATION(AL) ANALYSIS (or CA)

Conversation analysis is a form of systematic analysis which examines the use of ordinary language and asks how everyday conversation and interaction work. This type of inquiry focuses on **naturally occurring talk** (talk that is not especially set up for the research) and on the organisation and ordering of speech exchanges. While researchers primarily examine speech patterns, they also analyse non-verbal behaviour in interactions, such as facial expressions, gestures and other body language, as well as routine and rule-following behaviour. They uncover the structures behind 'talk-in-interaction' (Psathas, 1995) and investigate how conversation and interaction order are produced.

The origins of conversation analysis
CA was initially developed in the 1960s and 1970s in the United States by Harold Garfinkel, Harvey Sacks, Emmanuel Schegloff and others. While other types of discourse analysis have their roots in the field of linguistics, CA originates in *ethnomethodology* with elements of both sociology and *phenomenology*.

Ethnomethodology focuses, in particular, on the world of social practices, interactions and rules (Turner, 1974) and their underlying reality. Garfinkel attempted to demonstrate the ways in which members of society construct social reality and generate coherence and order.

Ethnomethodologists focus on the 'practical accomplishments' of societal members, seeking to demonstrate that these individuals make sense of their actions on the basis of 'tacit knowledge', their shared understanding of the rules of interaction and language.

The use of CA

CA focuses on what individuals say in their everyday talk and on their inter-actions. Through conversation, movement and gesture, we learn of people's intentions and ideas. The sequencing and turn-taking in conversations demonstrate the meaning individuals give to situations and show that they inhabit a shared world. Body movements too are the focus of analysis. Conversation analysts do not carry out interviews to collect *data* but analyse ordinary talk, 'naturally occurring' conversations. The sections of talk which they analyse are relatively small and the analysis is detailed. CA makes the assumption that talk is 'structurally organised' and each turn of talk is influenced by the context of what has gone on before and establishes a context towards which the next turn will be oriented. Like other qualitative researchers, conversation analysts attempt to examine the data without preformulated hypotheses or impositions.

CA is most often used in sociological or education studies and occasionally in health and social work research. Researchers generally audio- or video-tape these interactions and transcribe the conversations in a particular way, in a **notation system** largely developed by Gail Jefferson and described by Atkinson & Heritage (1984). The transcribing conventions contain symbols describing the characteristics of talk, such as intonation, pauses and emphases. These transcription procedures are necessary because of the detailed analysis and close *observation*. Even apparent trivialities are important. The transcription of tapes helps researchers understand the way in which the interaction order is constructed; indeed, it is often the first step in the discovery of particular features of talk and structure in interaction.

Researchers look for the sequential structure in interaction to uncover the nature of turn-taking. They have demonstrated, for instance, that speakers are oriented to each other; every person who speaks orients himself or herself to what the prior speaker has said immediately before. Each speech exchange is a **unit**.

There are a number of procedures which the researcher carries out. The investigation focuses particularly on opening and closing sequences. This includes speech used in telephone talk, compliments or greetings. Researchers, be they sociologists, anthropologists or linguists, examine work settings, such as medical settings or business situations. CA is also often used in communication research.

There are examples for CA which show how talk is generated and organised by people, and how it follows an orderly process in which a turn-taking system exists. Tapes show what actually takes place in a setting. The analysis of CA includes the discovery of regularities in speech or body movement, the search for deviant cases and the integration with other findings (Heritage, 1988). Conversation analysts emphasise the formal characteristics of interaction at the expense of content, but they do focus on the dynamic aspects in which inter-action takes place (Leudar & Antaki, 1988).

CA is difficult, highly complex and very detailed. Researchers may not find it easy, and one would not recommend it to novice researchers.

CO-OPERATIVE INQUIRY

Co-operative inquiry is a form of participative research in which a group (sometimes only consisting of two people) carry out collaborative research on an experience or 'aspect of the human condition' (Heron, 1996). This research is essentially phenomenological and focuses on the search for meaning in experiences.

Co-operative inquiry developed from articles, books and discussions by Reason and Heron and their colleagues during the 1970s and 1980s [for instance, Heron (1971); Reason (1988); and Reason & Rowan (1981)]. Peter Reason and his colleagues established a Centre for Action Research in Profes-sional Practice (CARPP) in 1994 in the School of Management, University of Bath. Heron again articulated the philosophy and strategies of co-operative inquiry in 1996 (Heron, 1996).

Co-operative inquiry is based on the belief that human beings have the fundamental right to autonomy and participation in decision-making about issues which affect them directly. Reason (1994: 1) calls it 'research *with* people rather than research *on* people'. Reason & Heron (1995) claim that people can investigate others when all the *participants* take part in decisions about the direction of the research. This includes the right to make decisions about research design, such as selecting ways of data generation, analysis and interpretation, and about the dissemination of results. The individuals facilitating the research and the other participants become **co-researchers**. For instance, nurse lecturers might wish to study the impact of gender on nursing. They can plan a study in collaboration with other nurses in which the nurses themselves make decisions about the *research design*, *data collection* and *data analysis*. This does mean that participants are first trained in the ways of co-operative inquiry.

The stages of the inquiry cycle in co-operative inquiry consist of reflection, action, full immersion and reflection (Heron, 1996).

The stages of the inquiry cycle

(1)   The first reflection phase is one in which co-researchers:
    choose the topic for inquiry
    make a statement about it
    develop a plan of action
    decide on a way of recording the experiences
(2)   The first action phase includes:
    exploring an experience or condition
    applying a range of inquiry skills
    recording the data
(3)   Full immersion involves:
    gaining insight and awareness
    'losing the way'
    going beyond the format of the research
(4)   The second reflection phase consists of:
    sharing experiences and reviewing the topic
    choosing an action plan for the next phase
    reviewing and modifying the ways of recording data

This cycle is followed by more cycles. Heron advises, but does not stipulate, five to eight full cycles until all the strands come together. This includes collaboration in writing a report if this is decided by the co-researchers.

COVERT RESEARCH

This is a research process in which researchers do not disclose their presence and identity as researchers, and *participants* have no knowledge of their research identity. Sometimes they even use concealed tape recorders. Covert research has been carried out in studies about the National Front, for instance (Fielding, 1981). Sometimes the justification is that nothing of interest or importance would be found if the research were overt, or that the situation could never be researched openly because researchers might not be granted permission to carry out the research. In health care, social work and educational settings, covert research is generally considered problematic and sometimes unethical. Indeed, one would have to debate whether it is appropriate in any situation.

CRITICAL INCIDENT TECHNIQUE

The critical incident technique is a type of data collection which focuses on people's behaviour in critical situations in order to solve problems in task performance. Researchers examine those events that are significant for a particular process. They collect examples of critical incidents in the situation under study, and participants give an account of the way in which they act in critical situations or times of crisis. Generally the researchers ask about the critical event and gain a perspective about effective and ineffective behaviour in specific decisive and important situations.

The critical incident technique was initially developed as a result of the Aviation Psychology Program in the United States to collect information from pilots about their behaviour when flying a mission. In particular, the psychologists asked for reports about critical incidents which helped or hindered the successful outcome of the mission. Through analysis of these reports, a list of components for successful performance was generated from the data.

Flanagan (1954) developed and refined the procedure for industrial psychology to assess the outcomes of task performance, in personnel selection and in identifying motivation and factors in effective counselling (Woolsey, 1986). Although the method was neglected after the 1950s, it can be a useful, effective and qualitative approach to studying critical events in order to improve task performance. Flanagan states that the technique is 'a procedure for gathering certain important facts concerning behaviour in defined situations'.

Woolsey (1986) lists four stages in the critical incident technique, whereas Cormack (1996) mentions six. The stages of both authors overlap:

(1)   The researchers decide on the aim of the research
(2)   They design and plan the research
(3)   The data are collected
(4)   The data are analysed

The stages of the critical incident technique

(1)   The first step consists of stating a clear aim; this will include choosing the type of events on which researchers wish to focus.

(2)   The second stage involves selecting a purposive sample from which to collect data. The sample size depends on the number of critical incidents, not on the number of people interviewed or observed.

(3)   Generally researchers collect the *data* through *observation* and focused or semi-structured *interviews*.

(4)   The data are analysed in a similar way to other qualitative data. There is, however, a slight difference. Researchers choose a stronger frame of reference in this type of research as they wish to focus on particular events.

The critical incident approach is very useful and relevant in particular for research in the professional arena such as teaching, medicine and nursing (Cormack (1996) quotes several examples for nursing, while Woolsey (1986) discusses it in counselling).

CRITICAL THEORY

Critical theory involves the belief that rational human beings are able to critically assess and change society and become emancipated. The theorists are critical of the 'scientific' version of truth and objective reality and stress the influence of 'values, judgments and interests of humankind' (Carr & Kemmis, 1986: 132). These ideas had their origin in Marxism and were developed initially by the Frankfurt School of Social Science and Jürgen Habermas, who states that critical social science has its place between philosophy and natural science.

Critical social research is based on this theory, and its result is a change in the lives of people which they initiate themselves through an understanding of their social condition. Critical *ethnography*, feminist standpoint research and some forms of *action research* and *phenomenology* are also influenced by the ideas of critical theory.

CROSS-GENDER INTERVIEW

A cross-gender *interview* is an interview in which men interview women or vice versa. These interviews have different conversation patterns and often generate *data* different from that derived from same-gender interviews (Rubin & Rubin, 1995). Both can be useful. Most feminists, however, believe that cross-gender interviews are inappropriate for a number of reasons. (See *feminist research*.)

The same issues arise when interviews across different classes or ethnic groups take place. As these types of interview are more difficult and might be influenced by a lack of mutual understanding between interviewer and *participant* (always a problem in interviews), immersion in the setting and reflexivity are essential for the researcher. However, researcher and participants cannot always be matched; even for practical reasons this is not possible. Who, for instance, would interview frail old people or children?

CULTURE

Culture can be defined as the total way of life of a group, the learnt behaviour that is socially constructed and transmitted. The life experiences of members of a cultural group include a communication system which they share. This consists of signs such as gestures, facial expressions and language, as well as cultural artefacts (all messages which the members of a culture recognise, and whose meaning they understand).

Anthropology is concerned with culture, and anthropologists immerse and involve themselves in cultures. The research method of anthropology is *ethnography*. Ethnographers analyse, compare and examine groups and their rules of behaviour. The relationship of individuals to the group and to each other is also explored. The study of change, in particular, helps ethnographers understand cultures and subcultures.

D

DATA

The data are the information that the researcher collects and in which the findings originate. In qualitative research they consist of words or actions of the *participants* which the researcher hears and observes. Qualitative data can also be text such as *fieldnotes* and journals, tape-recorded interviews, letters, diaries, or photographs and films. Historical documents are also sources of data.

Raw data can be divided into **unfiltered** and **filtered** data (Schwandt & Halpern, 1988). The term 'unfiltered data' refers to data not yet interpreted and those from which no inferences have been made. They are the data prior to reduction through *coding* and categorising. Filtered data are those from which some inferences have already been made. (See *data sources*.)

(Researchers using qualitative methods are clear that they mean words, actions, documents, etc., when they discuss data. The term qualitative data means something quite different when used in quantitative research. The term has traditionally referred to data which have a nominal or categorical scale of measurement (May *et al.*, 1990). This type of datum, for instance gender, type of therapy, etc., is coded numerically. The numerical codes assigned to the data are arbitrary and therefore do not have the usual meaning attached to quantitative data in terms of direct numerical relationship. Nominal data are therefore referred to as 'qualitative' to distinguish them from interval or ordinal data where the numerical codes have direct computational significance. This might help explain why quantitative researchers often expect qualitative researchers to quantify their 'qualitative' data.)

(Data is the plural of the Latin word datum – the given – but these days the term data is often used in the singular, especially in American texts.)

DATA ANALYSIS

Data analysis in *qualitative research* means breaking down the *data* and searching for codes and *categories* which are then reassembled to form themes. Data analysis takes place from the beginning of *data collection*. The focus becomes progressively clearer. In the data analysis the researcher revisits the aim and the initial research question. The process of analysis involves several steps.

(1)   Ordering and organising the collected material
(2)   Re-reading the data
(3)   Breaking the material into manageable sections
(4)   Identifying and highlighting meaningful phrases
(5)   Building, comparing and contrasting categories
(6)   Looking for consistent patterns of meanings
(7)   Searching for relationships and grouping categories together
(8)   Recognising and describing patterns, themes and typologies
(9)   Interpreting and searching for meaning

The data are scanned and organised from the very beginning of the study. If gaps and inadequacies occur, they can be filled by collecting more data or refocusing on the initial aims of the study. While this work goes on, researchers select particular aspects which they examine more closely than others, because they seem more important for the emerging ideas.

In re-reading the data, thoughts and observations can be recorded, and a search for regularities can begin. The first interview – or the first detailed description of observation – is scanned and marked off into sections of data which are then given codes: words or short sentences which contain the gist of the sentence or paragraph. The second and third interview transcripts are then analysed and compared with the first. Commonalities and similar codes are sorted and grouped together. That is, researchers look for recurrent ideas and consistent patterns in the data. This happens throughout data collection and analysis. Thematically similar sets are placed together. The researcher then tries to find the links between the categories and describes and summarises them. From this stage onwards diagrams are helpful because they present the links and patterns graphically. Regularities and sets of similar ideas are grouped into **categories** which the researcher compares and reduces to major constructs. Broad **patterns** of thought and behaviour emerge. The patterns and regularities have their basis in the actual observations and interviews; they will be linked to the categories and themes drawn from the literature.

The data analysis in different qualitative approaches is similar, though not necessarily the same. (See data analysis in *grounded theory* and *phenomenology*, for instance.)

Secondary data analysis – the analysis of other researchers' data – is also possible. It is not used much in qualitative research because one of the principles of the qualitative approach is the involvement of the researcher with the participants and the collection of secondary data does not, of course, involve the researcher and participants directly. Reinharz (1993) shows that researchers can, and occasionally do, analyse data collected by others.

DATA COLLECTION

Data collection involves the gathering of information for a research project through a variety of *data sources*. There should also be a plan for *recording* these data. Qualitative researchers sometimes reject the term 'collecting' data. They use instead 'generating' data (Mason, 1996) or even 'making' data (Koch, 1996). These terms sometimes seem suitable in qualitative approaches because researchers do not merely collect and describe data in a neutral and detached manner but are involved in a more creative way: 'the researcher is seen as actively constructing knowledge' (Mason, 1996: 36). Nevertheless, it should be clear that researchers do not 'make up' or invent these data.

DATA LOGGING

Data logging, according to Lofland & Lofland (1995), is the detailed recording and registering of data in interview *transcripts* and *fieldnotes* as well as the collection of documents and visual data such as films and photography. Researchers record all relevant information, even that which seems unimportant or trivial at the time of data collection.

DATA MANAGEMENT

Data management is the systematic task of handling data such as collecting, storing and retrieving (Miles & Huberman, 1994). This is planned prior to the research. It includes the organisation of data. Data will be on disc, on paper or on tape. A filing system will assist in managing data more easily.

DATA SOURCES

These are sources from which researchers extract their data. In qualitative research these may be ***interviews*** and **naturally occurring talk** such as discussions (for instance at meetings), conversations – including **telephone conversations**, *observations*, **photographs** and **films**, **diaries**, **letters** or **historical documents**. Some of these sources are contained in tapes or books. Other data sources could be meetings, job interviews or consultations in business or health care settings. Even paintings can be sources of data, particularly when used in a historical context.

Photographs are often included as data by anthropologists and historians. They can provide pictures of the culture or the era under study, but they are also useful for research into interaction – for instance interaction of teachers and students in classroom settings.

DEBRIEFING

Debriefing is the process of discussing the research process and reassuring participants after the research has finished. In qualitative health research with patients this is of particular importance, although the researcher is obliged to reassure participants in all types of research – particularly in research with sensitive topics. (See also *disengagement*)

DECONTEXTUALISATION

In qualitative research this means dividing data into segments and freeing them from their context. Researchers then **recontextualise** by organising and 'reassembling' the data and placing them back into context. Tesch (1990) uses this term in her discussion on computers in qualitative research. (See also *context*.)

DEDUCTION

Deduction means that researchers move from the general to the specific, that is, they start with a general theory from which a conclusion is deduced. Researchers then search for empirical evidence by testing a *hypothesis* through collecting data from observation and analysing them. The object of the analysis is to try to falsify the hypothesis (Popper, 1959) and establish probability. Deductive reasoning is often used in the natural sciences when the research starts, though by no means always. Glaser & Strauss (1967) advise against initial deductive reasoning for qualitative research because researchers who use this approach explore the theory derived from its founders rather than grounding theory in lived reality. (See also *induction*.)

DELIMITATION

The delimitation shows the **boundaries**, both physical and social, which limit the scope of the research (Cresswell, 1994). Researchers state these in the proposal and the write up. This demonstrates to the reader the confines of the research. The field may be small or large, but boundaries need to be set as the researcher decides what will or will not be studied in a particular project. The boundaries are in the control of the researchers and imposed by them but are also inherent in the research questions. In many types of qualitative research the delimitation might be changed during the process of the research so that new ideas or sampling units can be added, for instance in *grounded theory* because of theoretical sampling. (See also *limitation*.)

DIMENSIONAL ANALYSIS

This is a type of analysis used by Schatzman (1991) as a modification of *grounded theory* analysis. He claims that original GT lacks a structural basis and does not explain the detailed operations for generating theory (Kools *et al.*, 1996). Dimensional analysis assists in the process of making sense of interactions. The researcher engages with the data and selects the most significant and relevant dimensions which are the main concern of the participants. Dimensions are the elements of a phenomenon. The data are examined until enough dimensions have been considered to explain the phenomenon under study. These explanations form the main thread of the research, and they are significant. The perspective is the dimension most important to the emerging theoretical ideas and the one that has most explanatory power. Instead of adopting a linear view of the research process, researchers attempt to take multiple perspectives on a particular problem by searching for its dimensions. Schatzman adopts the 'cycle of inductive and deductive reasoning' (Robrecht, 1995). This type of analysis seems very similar to other forms of grounded theory.

DISCOURSE ANALYSIS

Discourse analysis (DA) in psychology is an analysis of text and language which draws on 'accounts' for action which participants present, and this type of discourse analysis has been carried out by psychologists. *Accounts* consist of forms of ordinary talk and reasoning of people, as well as other sources of text, such as historical documents, diaries, letters or reports. DA is not just a method but a specific approach to the social world and research (Potter, 1996a). It focuses on the construction of talk in social action. In common with other types of qualitative inquiry, discourse analysts initially use an inductionist approach by collecting and reviewing data before arriving at theories and general principles. As the structural analysis of discourse, DA is often used in media and communication research (van Dijk, 1985) to analyse 'message data'. An example would be an analysis of the speeches of politicians. Language itself, and reality, are socially constructed. The way people use language and text is taken for granted within a culture (Gill, 1996).

It is important to read the documents and transcripts carefully before interpreting them. The first step in the analysis is a verbatim transcription of the interview and a close look at other documents. The relevant documents are read and re-read until researchers have become familiar with the data. Immersion in the data, after all, is a trait of all qualitative research. Important issues and themes can then be highlighted. The analysis proceeds like other *qualitative research*; analysts code the *data*, look for relationships and search for patterns and regularities which generate tentative *hypotheses*. Through the process, they always take the context into account and generate analytical notes (see *memoing*).

Like other qualitative research, the findings from discourse analysis are not generalisable. Indeed researchers are not concerned with generalisability, because the analysis is based on language and text in a specific social context. There are a number of similarities between *conversation analysis* and discourse analysis; both CA and DA focus on language and text. Whereas DA generally considers the broader context, CA emphasises turn-taking and explains the deeper sense of interaction in which people are engaged, particularly 'naturally occurring' talk, while discourse analysts look mainly at interview material, although they can also use records, newspaper articles or reports of meetings, etc.

Discourse analysts are interested in the ways through which social reality is constructed in interaction and action. DA is based on the belief that language does not just mirror the world of social members and cultures but also helps to construct it. Indeed there are not just one but many 'languages' (Banister *et al.*, 1994). Potter & Wetherell (1987) and Potter (1996b: 130, 131) developed the notion of 'interpretative repertoires' which they see as a set of related concepts 'organised around one or more central metaphors'. These provide researchers with common-sense concepts of a group or a culture. Language is 'action oriented'; it is used so people can 'do'. It is shaped by the cultural and social context in which it occurs. Social groups possess a variety of repertoires and use them appropriately in different situations. The integrated discourses of people about various specific areas in their lives generate a text (Banister *et al.*, 1994). Discourse analysts must therefore be aware of the context in which action takes place so that the context too can be analysed. The same text can be interpreted in different ways: different versions of reality exist in different contexts. The discourse analysis of psychologists and linguists focuses on text. Readers can make judgements about this type of research because they themselves possess knowledge of everyday discourse and its construction.

McHoul & Grace (1995) differentiate between Foulcauldian and non-Foucauldian discourse. Michel Foucault, the French historian and philosopher, made the concept of discourse famous while describing the links of language with disciplines and institutions. For him, discourses are bodies of knowledge, by which he means both academic scholarship and institutions, which exist in disciplines. Indeed, he claims that discourse reproduces institutions. Social phenomena are constructed through language. Specific language is connected with specialist fields, for instance 'professional discourse', 'scientific discourse' or 'medical discourse'. In Foucault's works, discourses as specialist languages are linked to power. Discourse analysis discovers the language which operates within the particular discourse under study. For instance, professionals use particular types of discourse to impose their own or the official version of reality on their clients.

DISENGAGEMENT

Disengagement is the state that researchers need to achieve when they finish their research and 'leave the field'. This happens when nothing new can be learnt. Researchers start distancing themselves from both the setting and the people in it. They negotiate with *participants* and *gatekeepers* the best ways of 'getting out'. In qualitative research this is not always as easy as in other types of research because of greater immersion and engagement. The closer relationship with participants, too, makes disengagement more difficult as they might have relied on the researcher to provide a listening post. In research in the health care field this may even mean that the participants used the interviewer for therapeutic reasons. Researchers need empathy, tact and diplomacy to leave some field settings.

DISSEMINATION

Dissemination of research means that the research is made public to other researchers and those in the practice situation who apply it. There are a number of ways to do this: researchers write reports for the appropriate agencies, as well as books or articles in relevant professional or academic journals. They present research papers at conferences or disseminate the research informally at meetings or chance encounters with others who are interested in it. The writer or speaker has to remember to address the audience for whom the specific book, article or talk is intended. He or she also explains why the discussion of this problem is significant for the audience and what its implications are for professional practice. The best way for academics to disseminate research is to write articles for refereed and high-status journals for the academic community. For dissemination to practitioners, articles in widely read, popular, professional journals are useful because they address the largest possible audience.

DOCUMENTARY SOURCES

Documentary data can be text-based or non-text-based (Mason, 1996), consisting of written documents and records as well as graphic presentations and photographs or films. Researchers use these because they give information about situations which cannot be investigated by direct observation or questioning (Hammersley & Atkinson, 1995). Documents consist typically of personal diaries, letters, autobiographies and biographies but also of official documents and reports; they range from informal documentary sources to formal and official reports such as newspapers or minutes of meetings. Timetables, case notes and reports can become the focus of the investigation. The researcher treats them like transcriptions of interviews or detailed descriptions of observations, that is, they are coded and categorised. By acting as sensitising devices they make researchers aware of important issues. Many of these texts have been in existence for decades or centuries – for instance historical documents – whereas others are initiated and organised by the researchers themselves. Historical documents, archives and products of the media exist independently from researchers while personal diaries might be written through their intervention or instigation. Researchers who carry out *historical research* also use documentary sources.

Scott (1990) differentiates between types of document by referring to them as **closed**, **restricted**, **open-archival** and **open-published**. Access to closed documents is limited to a few people, namely their authors and those who commissioned them. As far as restricted documents are concerned, researchers can only gain access with the permission of insiders under particular conditions.

Permission for access needs to be obtained from the living authors of diaries and keepers of other confidential documents. Open-archival documents are available to any person, subject to administrative conditions and opening hours of libraries and archives. Published documents, of course, can be accessed by anybody at any time.

Qualitative researchers most often seek access to diaries – people's own accounts of their lives – and letters, but also to historical documents or the products of the media. Merriam (1988) points out the non-reactivity of documentary data. They do not change through the presence of the researcher but are grounded in their context, and this makes them useful and rich sources of information for researchers. Some researchers encourage *participants* to keep a diary for analysis rather than analysing existing diaries.

Through documents, professionals who carry out research, for instance in nursing, teaching and social work, acquire a perspective on history which gives them insiders' views on past lives and attitudes. On the other hand, they can analyse contemporary documents – such as articles and comments in the press – and become aware of the significant features of issues or the dramatisation of particular events. Last, and most importantly, professionals can trace the perspectives of diary or autobiography writers by collecting, reading and analysing these personal documents. Through these procedures researchers can gain knowledge about the experiences of others in a particular context and at a particular time.

The documentary sources are not viewed uncritically. Researchers are concerned about four major criteria which determine the quality of the documents: authenticity, credibility, representativeness and meaning (Scott, 1990). To demonstrate authenticity for historical documents, questions about their *context* as well as their writers' intentions and biases must be asked. Often they involve official accounts written for publication. Credibility, too, involves some of these questions. Accuracy might be affected by the writers' proximity in time and place and the conditions under which the information was acquired. Representativeness of documents is difficult to prove because researchers often have no information on the numbers or variety of documents about a particular event.

Scott claims that the most significant aim of the document collection and analysis is their meaning and interpretation. It is easier to analyse a personal contemporary document with familiar language and context than to assess the representativeness or authenticity of a historical document whose context can only be assumed. Therefore, the researcher can only try to interpret the meaning of the text in context, study the situation and conditions in which it is written and try to establish the writer's intentions.

As in other types of data, the meaning is tentative and provisional only and may change when new data present a challenge and demand reappraisal. Hammersley & Atkinson (1995) warn that documents may generate *bias* as they were often written by and for élites or people in power. That in itself, however, can be useful because these documents, too, disclose beliefs and ideologies of particular people in a particular time and location.

DOMAIN

A domain is 'a category of cultural meaning that includes other smaller categories' (Spradley, 1980: 88) or an organised unit. The term is used in *ethnography*. All cultures have these categories which are clusters and classifications characterised by semantic relationships. Spradley differentiates between three types of domain: **folk domains**, which come from the language of ordinary people in the culture under investigation; **mixed domains** which stem from the vocabulary of both researcher and *participants*; and **analytic domains**, which include researchers' terms and theoretical concepts. The researcher searches for 'cover terms'; Spradley gives examples: an oak is a kind of tree or a parent is a kind of teacher. Domain analysis, a step in ethnographic analysis, explores the way cultural members use shared understanding reflected in the use of language. Ethnographers search for patterns within a *culture* and identify these shared cultural meanings.

DROSS RATE

The dross rate is the amount of information from *participants* that is irrelevant for the outcome of the research in hand. This rather contemptuous term should not be used too much as none of the information from the participants is seen as dross by them, and may indeed be significant for their own lives. However, most researchers have an agenda within which they have to work, and this means that they cannot include everything. They should always examine carefully which elements of an interview or diary are 'dross' so that they do not discard important data.

E

ELITE INTERVIEW

An élite interview is an *interview* with particularly powerful, wealthy or high-status people. In their relations with the *participants* qualitative researchers have to overcome their awe (or indeed their negative feelings). Researchers more often research low status or powerless people for a variety of reasons such as easier access and greater interest.

EMICS

This is a term with a variety of definitions, meanings and applications. Coined by Pike (1954), a linguist, it was later taken up by the anthropologist Harris (1976). It became widely used in *ethnography* and other qualitative inquiry where it often takes a different meaning from the one originally given.

The **emic** perspective is the insider's or 'native's' perception – to use its simplest explanation – while the **etic** perspective is the imposed framework of the researcher and outsider. In social and anthropological research this means that a distinction is made between the 'subjective' knowledge of the participant and the 'scientific' knowledge of the social scientist. The insiders' accounts of reality produce knowledge of the reasons why people act as they do. In the early days of ethnography, for instance, the anthropologist Malinowski (1922) focused on the 'native's' point of view to find out about the reasons for behaviour. A researcher who uses the emic perspective gives explanations of events from the cultural members' point of view and from inside their framework. For instance, when health professionals wish to examine the culture of patients, they use not only the perceptions of nurses or doctors but also those of the patients themselves. This perspective of cultural members is important in qualitative inquiry, particularly at the start, as it prevents the imposition of the values and beliefs from the culture of researchers to other cultures. The researchers who examine a culture or subculture gain knowledge of the existing rules and patterns from its members; the emic perspective is thus culturally specific. It corresponds with the reality and definition of informants, and emic categories are conceptual patterns derived from the members' information in the culture under study. (The long and complex debate of emics and etics cannot be developed here, but interested readers might follow the discussion in Headland *et al.*, 1990.)

ENTRY (or ENTRÉE)

Entry means access to the research setting. When researchers select a site, they also have to negotiate entry and *access* to this setting and contact the participants in it. They need the co-operation of both participants and *gatekeepers* for entry.

EPIPHANY

This term, which in the Christian religion means the appearance of Jesus to the Magi, is used by Denzin (1989a). He sees 'epiphany' as a significant moment in people's lives that often changes them profoundly. Qualitative researchers record and use the stories participants tell about these critical points in their lives.

EPISTEMOLOGY

Epistemology is the theory of knowledge. Epistemological considerations depend on beliefs about the nature of knowledge. Knowledge forms and communications of knowledge to others are important for qualitative researchers. Hitchcock & Hughes (1995) suggest that assumptions about forms of knowledge, access to knowledge and ways of acquiring knowledge are epistemological issues. All this has an influence on the research process including data collection and analysis.

ESRC

This is the abbreviated form of the Economic and Social Research Council, a British research council which funds research in the social sciences including qualitative research. (Formerly this was called the Social Science Research Council, SSRC.)

ETHICS

Ethics in research relates to moral standards. Ethical concerns have to be considered in all research methods and at each stage of the *research design*. For instance, ethical issues are important in relation to the aim or the *research questions*. Researchers apply the principles that protect the *participants* in the research from harm or risk and follow ethical guidelines and legal rules. The rights of the individuals are that they are not to be harmed, that they give their consent on the basis of information and knowledge about the research, that their participation is voluntary, and that the researcher follows the rules of confidentiality and anonymity (Couchman & Dawson, 1995).

Respect for autonomy means that the participants in the research must make an independent and informed choice without coercion. The good derived from the research must be weighed against the potential risk, and the benefits must outweigh the risks for the individual and the wider society. The principle of justice implies that the research strategies and procedures are fair and just.

The concern with ethical issues emerged initially from risky and harmful biomedical research with human 'subjects' in Hitler's Germany which eventually led to the Nuremberg Code (1949). This gave guidelines for research and stated that individuals have to give voluntary consent to any research in which they participate before it can proceed. The principles of ethical research were followed up and re-established after some dangerous research was carried out in the US on people with learning difficulties, and on patients and prisoners without their knowledge or consent. The 'Declaration of Helsinki' was taken on by the World Health Organization in 1964 and extended in 1975. Now firmly established ethical codes exist, particularly for medical and nursing research but also in other caring professions, in business and in academic research.

Ethical problems

Qualitative researchers have to consider a variety of issues:

❑ Researchers explore the inner feelings and thoughts of the participants who are clients, colleagues or other professionals, and they have to act with sensitivity and diplomacy
❑ Informed consent is problematic as participants cannot be fully informed at the very beginning because of the tentative and exploratory nature of qualitative research
❑ The informants' anonymity might be threatened by the detailed description of the research process, the data and the sample

❏   The vulnerable position of clients and their feelings of obligation might prevent them from refusing participation in the research although they may wish to do so
❏   The researcher, who is part of a profession or an organisation, has conflicting role expectations as investigator and professional
❏   Participants do not always comprehend the research role of professionals who also have a professional role
❏   Individuals may become fearful and distressed during interviews
❏   Over-involvement and empathy could produce assumptions and inaccuracies in the research
❏   *Ethics committees* do not always fully understand the character of qualitative research

Informed consent and voluntary participation

Informed, voluntary consent is an explicit agreement by the research participants, given without threat or inducement, based on information which any reasonable person would want to receive before consenting to participate (Sieber, 1992).

Qualitative researchers have inherent problems with *informed consent*. When the research starts, they have no specific objectives, though they may have general aims or a focus. The nature of qualitative research is its flexibility. Surprising ideas often arise during data collection and may take researchers in unexpected directions. Qualitative research focuses on the meanings and interpretation of the participants. The researcher develops ideas that are grounded in the data rather than testing previously constructed hypotheses. Therefore, the researcher is not able to inform research participants of the exact path of the research, and informed consent is not a once-and-forever permission but goes on as the research proceeds.

The process of informed consent is set firmly within the principle of respect for autonomy. This principle demands that participation is voluntary and that informants are aware not only of the benefits of the research but also of the risks they take. First-time researchers, in particular, should take care that there is no major risk, though all research involves some dangers. Participants must be informed throughout about the voluntary nature of participation in research and about the possibility to withdraw at any stage.

It is useful to anticipate potential problems in the course of the research and consider their solutions. The researcher must be aware that the research might threaten participants, superiors or institutions, even if it is intended to have a positive effect. There may also be conflict between the recognition of individuals' rights and the wish to advance knowledge and gain information.

The researcher should try to be as clear as possible in stating the demands on the time of the participants and about the general direction of the research so that they can agree or refuse to take part on the basis of information about it. Sometimes this might be difficult as the status of a researcher could prevent participants from giving honest, open and non-biased answers.

Anonymity in research means that the participants in the process cannot be identified at any time by the reader of the report. When researchers gain *access* to participants, they generally promise anonymity. This is more difficult to achieve in qualitative research than in other approaches, and individuals are more easily identifiable to others due to longer, more intimate involvement and quotes from interviews.

Researchers protect the anonymity of participants through the following means:

(1) The pseudonyms used have no resemblance to the real name of the participants.

(2) Researchers take care that informants cannot be identified by gender, age or ethnic group membership unless this is a feature of the research and previously discussed. The danger exists in studies where only one or two participants belong to a particular age, gender or ethnic group. Concerning age, researchers can protect individuals by changing the age of all informants by a number of years (for instance they can change ages systematically by two years). Researchers need to state that they have changed the ages of the participants without disclosing the number of years. If disclosure of group membership is essential for the research, care must be taken that informants cannot be recognised. The occupation of participants too, should only be stated if this is important for the research.

(3) Names are not linked to the data. Researchers identify informants on tapes and transcripts by number, letters or pseudonyms. Numbers and names are kept separate.

(4) Specific locations should not be named unless researchers make this explicit to the participants. For instance, instead of writing 'The research took place in the Nosmasten Hospital in Winchingham, Southshire', it could state 'The research took place in a small community hospital in the South of England'.

Confidentiality relates to the data and what can be done with them.

Participants often disclose private and personal information that they wish to keep confidential. This happens particularly in qualitative research because of its more intensive nature.

Generally researchers agree to the following with the participants. They must respect participants' wishes for the confidentiality of disclosures they do not wish to make public. As qualitative research relies on the use of quotes, participants must be informed that some of their words will be used. This can only be done with their permission.

Researchers assure the participants that only they and certain other, specified individuals have access to tapes and transcripts. Supervisors in academic research or typists might be exceptions, but they too should be briefed by researchers about the absolute confidentiality of the research. Researchers make sure that the data cannot be linked to specific informants and should not contain their real names and identities.

Children, people with learning difficulties, and those who have a mental or terminal illness need particular protection, and so do very frail and elderly individuals. Researchers are obliged to ask the parents or legal guardians for permission to research with children and individuals with learning difficulties, although the participants themselves must also be asked. Research with vulnerable groups should only be carried out by experienced researchers after careful consideration.

Researchers ask potential participants for permission to interview or observe, stating clearly the right of refusal or withdrawal and assuring confidentiality. In research with children, the assent of parents and of the children themselves must be obtained. If researchers are not known to potential participants, they introduce themselves by name and identify their institution. It is useful to carry a short letter of introduction from the institution.

Practical considerations

Consent forms are given or sent to participants for signature. The form gives the aim and outline of the research and describes briefly the implications for the informants. The consent form should not be too long and must be clearly expressed in plain English, not in technical terminology or jargon. The signing of a consent form is not universally practised, and many participants only give their verbal consent.

Researchers do not always ask for written consent in circumstances where it is unduly difficult to obtain or intrusive. Written consent may prejudice the study or interfere with the researcher–participant relationship by formalising it. In researching colleagues, too, the written consent form is often seen as unnecessary. However, researchers should be aware that some ethics committees insist on a consent form.

When the main steps have been taken, the research can begin, always taking into account appropriate timing, site and situation.

ETHICS COMMITTEE

An ethics committee consists of a group of professional and lay people who scrutinise any research project that involves patients or clients or their relatives. Generally the ethics committee is attached to a Health Trust, but universities often have ethics committees too. Researchers fill out the ethics submission form of the relevant committee and send it for approval and consent. For research with clients, it does not suffice to obtain permission from immediate superiors, managers, peers (or consultants or general practitioners). Any piece of research in health care that deals with sensitive issues might aim for approval from the ethics committee, even if it involves colleagues rather than clients.

Members of committees are not always aware of the complex issues and dilemmas in all research methods. They are used to proposals in the field of biomedical, experimental research or surveys with large numbers of respondents and random sampling. For the qualitative researchers this means filling out and presenting ethics forms clearly and making a detailed statement of methods and procedures to the committee. Sometimes the committee demands a 'questionnaire'. The qualitative researcher must then send an interview guide with the type of questions that might be asked. Ethics committees sometimes call on researchers to explain and defend their research.

ETHNOGRAPHY

Ethnography is the research method of *anthropology*. An ethnography is the direct description of a *culture* or subculture.

As the oldest of the qualitative methods, ethnography has been used since ancient times, for instance in the descriptions of Greeks and Romans who wrote about the cultures which they encountered in their travels and wars. Deriving from the Greek, the term ethnography means a description of the people, literally 'writing of culture' (Atkinson, 1992). It can be distinguished from other forms of qualitative research by its emphasis on culture. In the early days of anthropology, ethnographers studied foreign and exotic settings but now they often focus on their own culture. Ethnographic data collection takes place mainly through *observations*, *interviews* and examination of documents.

Ethnographers stress the importance of studying human behaviour in the context of a culture in order to gain an understanding of the cultural phenomena, rules and norms. Agar (1990) explains that the meaning of ethnography is ambiguous; it refers both to a process (the methods and strategies of research) and to a product, the written story which is the outcome of the inquiry. People 'do' ethnography: they study a culture, observe its members' behaviours and listen to them. They also produce an ethnography, a written text.

Through ethnography researchers become culturally sensitive and identify the social influences on the individuals and groups they study. Hammersley & Atkinson (1995) claim that ethnographers aim to produce knowledge rather than apply this knowledge to professional practice, but much ethnography in education or in the health professions, for instance, is specifically intended to improve practice.

History and origins of ethnography

Modern ethnography emerged in particular in the 1920s and 1930s when famous anthropologists such as Malinowski (1922), Boas (1928) and Mead (1935), while searching for cultural patterns and rules, explored a variety of non-western cultures and the life ways of the people within them. When tribal groups were thought to be likely to disappear, researchers who wished to preserve aspects of vanishing cultures lived with them and wrote about them.

Initially these anthropologists explored only 'primitive' cultures (a term that demonstrates the patronising stance of many early anthropologists). When cultures became more linked with each other, and western anthropologists could not find homogeneous isolated cultures abroad, they turned to research their own cultures, acting as 'cultural strangers', that is, trying to see it from outside: everything is looked at with the eyes of an outsider. Sociologists, too, adopted ethnographic methods, immersing themselves in the culture or subculture in which they took an interest. Van Maanen (1988: 21) states that 'anthropologists go elsewhere to practise their trade while sociologists stay at home'; the distinction between these two groups is not so clear now. Experienced ethnographers and sociologists who are researching their own society take a new perspective on that which is already familiar. This approach to a familiar culture helps ethnographers not to take assumptions about their own society or cultural group for granted.

The *Chicago School* of sociology had an influence on later ethnographic methods because its members examined marginal cultural and 'socially strange' subcultures like the slums, ghettos and gangs of the city. A good example is the study by Whyte (1943) who investigated the urban gang subculture in an American city. *Street Corner Society* became a classic, and other sociologists used this work as a model for their own writing.

Sarantakos (1994) and Thomas (1993) distinguish between two types of ethnographic methods:

❏   descriptive or conventional ethnography
❏   critical ethnography

Descriptive ethnography focuses on the description of cultures or groups and, through analysis, uncovers patterns, typologies and categories. **Critical ethnography** involves the study of macro-social factors such as power, and examines common-sense assumptions and hidden agendas. It is meant to generate change in the setting it investigates or in the researcher who studies it. It is therefore more political (Thomas, 1993). Most kinds of ethnography use the same methods of analysis.

The main features of ethnography
The main features of ethnography are:

(1)   the collection of data from observation and interviews
(2)   *thick description* and the naturalistic stance
(3)   work with *key informants*
(4)   the *emic/etic* dimension

Researchers collect data by standard methods, mainly through observation and interviewing, but they also rely on documents such as letters, diaries and taped oral histories of people in a particular group or connected with it. Wolcott (1994) calls these strategies 'experiencing' (participant observation), 'enquiring' (interviewing), and 'examining' (studying documents).

As in other qualitative approaches, the researcher is the major research tool. Direct participant observation is the main way of collecting data from the culture under study. Observers try to become part of the culture, taking note of everything they see and hear, but they also interview members of the culture to gain their interpretations. The participants and their actions are observed, as are the ways in which they interact with each other. Special events and crises, the site itself and the use of space and time are also examined. Observers study the rules of a culture or subculture and the change that occurs over time in the setting. Observations become starting points for in-depth interviews. The researchers may not understand what they see, and ask the members of the group or culture to explain it to them. Participants then share their interpretations of events, rules and roles with the interviewer. Some of the interviews are formal and structured, but often researchers ask questions on the spur of the moment and have informal conversations with members. Often they uncover discrepancies between words and actions which become part of the analysis. Ethnographers take part in the life of people. They listen to their informants' interpretations of their actions. In essence, this involves a partnership between the investigator and the informants.

One of the major characteristics is **thick description**, a term that the anthropologist Geertz (1973) borrowed from the philosopher Ryle. It is description which makes explicit the detailed patterns of cultural and social relationships and puts them in *context*. Thick description must be theoretical and analytical in that researchers concern themselves with the abstract and general patterns and traits of social life in a culture.

As in other qualitative research, ethnographers generally use **purposive sampling**. This means ethnographers adopt certain criteria to choose a specific group and setting to be studied. The criteria for *sampling* must be explicit and systematic (Hammersley & Atkinson, 1995). Researchers should choose key informants carefully to make sure that they are suitable and representative of the group under study. Key informants often participate by informally talking about the cultural conduct or customs of the group. They become active collaborators in the research rather than passive respondents.

Ethnographers use the constructs of the informants and apply their own scientific conceptual framework, the so-called **emic** and **etic** perspectives (Harris, 1976). The insiders' accounts of reality help to uncover knowledge of the reasons why people act as they do.

There is a continuum between large- and small-scale studies, i.e. macro- and micro-ethnographies. Micro-ethnographies focus on subcultures or small settings. A macro-ethnography examines a larger culture with its institutions, communities and value systems. The large scope of study means a long period of time in the setting and often the work of several researchers.

'Doing' and writing an ethnography

The term *fieldwork* is used by ethnographers and other qualitative researchers to describe data collection outside laboratories. Ethnographers gain most of their data through fieldwork that involves mainly observation and interviewing. Fieldwork in *qualitative research* means working in the natural setting of the informants' culture, observing them and talking to them over prolonged periods of time. It aims to uncover patterns and regularities which the members of the culture can recognise. This is necessary so that informants get used to the researcher and behave naturally rather than 'putting on a performance'.

The best method of *data collection* in ethnographic research is **participant observation** – complete immersion in a culture or subculture. Researchers also rely on documents such as letters, diaries and the oral history of people in the culture they study. This includes noting down fleeting impressions as well as accurate and detailed descriptions of events and behaviour in *context*. While writing notes and describing what occurs in the situation, ethnographers become reflective and analytic.

Spradley (1979) lists four different types of fieldnotes in ethnography:

❑   the condensed account
❑   the expanded account
❑   the fieldwork journal
❑   analysis and interpretation notes

Condensed accounts are short descriptions made in the field during data collection whereas expanded accounts extend the descriptions and fill in detail. Ethnographers extend the short account as soon as possible after observation or interview if they were unable to record during data collection. In the fieldwork journal, ethnographers note their own biases, reactions and problems during fieldwork. Researchers use additional ways to record events and behaviour such as tapes, films or photographs, flowcharts and diagrams.

An ethnography consists of description, analysis and interpretation. Ethnographers describe what they see and hear while studying a culture and its members; they identify its main features and uncover relationships between them through analysis; they interpret the findings by asking for meaning and inferring it from the data. Researchers use **description** by writing a story which is a report of the actions, interactions and events within a cultural group. The reader should get a sense of the setting or 'a feel' for it and understand 'what's going on here'. The description is enhanced by the description of critical events, rituals or roles.

Data analysis entails working with the data. After processing them by coding, they are transformed from the raw data by the recognition of patterns and themes and linkages between ideas. Analysis brings order to disorderly data, and the researchers must show how they arrived at the structures and linkages. The analysis must accurately reflect the data. The findings have to be related back to the data to see whether there is a fit between them and the analytic *categories* and *themes*.

Researchers take the last step, that of **interpretation** during and after the analysis, making inferences, providing meaning and giving explanations for the phenomena. While researchers describe and analyse, they interpret the findings and gain insight in order to give meaning to them. Interpretation, although linked to analysis, is not as factual and is more speculative, involving theorising and explaining. Interpretation links the emerging ideas derived from the analysis to established theories through comparing and contrasting others' work with one's own. Eventually the story is put together from the descriptions, analyses and interpretations. It forms a coherent **storyline**.

Van Maanen (1988) uses the term 'tales' when discussing ethnographic writing. He differentiates mainly between (1) **realist tales**, (2) **confessional tales**, and (3) **impressionist tales** (although he also mentions others).

(1)   The traditional realist tale cut the ethnographer from the text and was written in the third person to give the ethnography a flavour of neutrality and objectivity. It focused on the mundane details of cultural life and generated the 'native's' point of view, the ordinary ways of life and routines of the informants. It lacked *reflexivity* and relied on only one interpretation, that of the author. Becker *et al.* (1961) are writers in the realist mode. In recent years, realist tales have become more personalised and self-reflexive, and are more often written using the *first person*, 'I'.

(2)   Confessional tales are written in very personal language which describes in detail the techniques and strategies in the field. Writers tell how they gained the knowledge presented in the ethnography, thus demonstrating the 'respectability' and disciplined nature of the fieldwork. The confessions of the authors show awareness of their own stance and biases. The writing of the tale is often stimulated when researchers experience surprise or shock in the fieldwork or through mistakes that occurred and caused problematic situations. Van Maanen stresses that authors of confessional tales usually confirm what they have done and try to demonstrate the adequacy of their work. Confessional tales have been more common in the last two decades. Examples of confessional tales are presented in Shaffir & Stebbins (1991). Realist and confessional tales are now often published in parallel or sequentially.

(3)   Impressionist tales are intended to present the culture under study in a creative and imaginative way. Authors attempt to pull the readers into the

story and reveal the developing *storyline* through which they learn about the culture gradually. The people inhabiting these stories are given names and personalities while their actions are described. The fieldworker-and-author has a place in the impressionist tale. Impressionist tales, according to van Maanen, are literary, artistic and contextual. He claims that some of the best ethnographies are written in the impressionist style.

Problems

There are a number of problems with ethnographic research. It is difficult to examine one's own group and become a '**cultural stranger**', questioning the assumptions of the familiar culture whose rules and norms have been internalised. Researchers often make statements that seem to be applicable to a whole range of similar situations, but an ethnography – like other qualitative research – cannot simply be generalised. Findings from one subculture or one setting are not automatically applicable to other settings.

ETHNOMETHODOLOGY

Ethnomethodology is a direction in sociology whose originator is the American sociologist, Harold Garfinkel (1967). It was developed by writers such as Schegloff, Sacks, Turner and Jefferson in the 1960s and 1970s. It is the exploration of 'ethnomethods' (peoples' or members' methods) and uncovers how members of society 'do' social life, share their reality and make sense of the world. Garfinkel and his colleagues criticise other sociologists for giving their own views rather than the ideas of the ordinary member of society. Social actors base their actions on **commonsense knowledge** which is learnt through socialisation processes and provides recipes for action. It is the practical knowledge which human beings have, but they do not always know that they possess it.

Ethnomethodology focuses on the world of social practices, in particular on interactions and interaction rules (Turner, 1974). Garfinkel demonstrated how members of society construct social reality by using 'common sense' methods to explain the world to themselves and others. Ethnomethodologists examine the 'practical accomplishments' of members of society, seeking to show that they make sense of their actions on the basis of *tacit knowledge*, their shared understanding of the rules of interaction and language.

The research method in ethnomethodology is *conversation analysis* (CA), although the term ethnomethodology itself is also used. Ethnomethodology is related to *symbolic interactionism*. Many concepts which were developed by

George Herbert Mead and other symbolic interactionists have influenced ethnomethodology, and interaction is its prime focus. Human beings are seen as active and creative. Watson & Seiler (1992: xiv) claim that even facts 'are not encountered ... but rather continuously constructed'.

ETHNONURSING

This is a term made popular by Leininger (1985) to describe the use of *ethnography* in nursing. She developed this as a modification and extension of ethnography. As in other ethnographic methods, ethnonursing deals with studies of a culture but it is also about nursing care and specifically generates nursing knowledge. Those who study ethnonursing aim to understand nursing and patient culture and attempt to advance clinical practice; for instance an oncology nurse could develop a research project about the culture of care in oncology.

ETHNOSCIENCE

Ethnoscience is a type of *ethnography* linked to linguistic forms and patterns. Ethnoscientists attempt to grasp cultural concepts and categories through the analysis of language and to comprehend their meaning in the context of a culture. They work with taxonomies that show relationships between concepts. Ethnoscience has its origin in the 1960s and 1970s when anthropologists wished to make their research more scientific. It is specifically used by Spradley (1970, 1979) and Werner & Schoepfle (1987).

ETICS

This is the outsider's or observer's perspective, the scientific point of view. (See also *emics*.)

EVALUATION RESEARCH

This research is a form of inquiry in which researchers judge a programme, a treatment or a practice for its success, effectiveness and efficiency. Many evaluation researchers use qualitative approaches. Qualitative evaluation researchers generally base their findings on interviews and observations as well as other evidence, and they analyse these data qualitatively (Patton, 1987, 1990). Evaluation resembles *action research* in the sense that the practices under study may be changed as an outcome of the research because evaluators not only make judgements but also disclose their findings to the relevant target group that has commissioned the research, and they might make recommendations for change. The evaluation proceeds in a similar way to other qualitative research:

❏ Researchers develop the research question
❏ They set the aims for the study
❏ They choose a sample
❏ They access gatekeepers and participants
❏ They collect and analyse the data
❏ They communicate and disseminate results
❏ They make recommendations

An example of evaluation research: a special course or curriculum is established for health or social care professionals. Researchers can evaluate the course itself and its quality or the effectiveness of the course. A teacher training programme can be evaluated and the results of the evaluation might change the programme.

F

FACESHEET

A facesheet is the first sheet of an interview transcript containing information about the interview and the participant such as date and place of interview, *pseudonym*, code or number of the interview, and the participant's gender, occupation or any other relevant facts.

The facesheet helps researchers to remember the details of the interview. Although the facesheet has its place at the top of the transcript and the researchers obtain the factual information as a warm-up for the interview, it is not always elicited from the participant and logged until the end of the interview.

Interviewers sometimes add a comment sheet in which they make notes on any specifics of the interview such as feelings and relationships and on the non-verbal behaviour of the participant. Generally, however, these comments become part of the *fieldnotes* in the diary.

FEMINIST RESEARCH

Feminist research is research that focuses on the experience and perception of women. Feminist approaches do not prescribe methods of analysing research but suggest ways of thinking about it. The intention is to make women visible, raise their consciousness and empower them. The most common form of feminist research is the *narrative* or *life history*, because it gives women the chance to tell their own stories in their own way, 'letting the women speak'. Because *qualitative research* has an affinity with the ideas of feminists, it is used more often than quantitative approaches (although they also see the latter as valid). Feminist research and *co-operative inquiry* share many of their most important features.

Some feminists believe in a separate and distinctive feminist research methodology, and consider that this type of inquiry is not merely a variation or branch of qualitative research (Stanley & Wise, 1993). Many researchers (for instance Harding, 1987) maintain that a distinctive feminist method does not exist, but that feminist researchers address certain epistemological and methodological issues related to gender.

The methodology gives women the opportunity to voice their concerns and interests, and is not merely concerned with the technical details of data analysis. The latter depends on the field in which researchers work and on the specific research question, although methods, too, reflect the feminist principles of equality between researcher and participant and focus on women's experiences and their empowerment. Taking into account the requirements of feminist research, researchers use *grounded theory*, *ethnography* and other types of *data analysis*. The focus on the 'lived experience' and the affective elements in the participants' lives means that phenomenological approaches are often taken in feminist qualitative research.

The term 'feminist standpoint research' is now frequently used. It is a less specific term than feminist methodology which carries with it the implication that feminist research uses a specific type of analysis. Feminist standpoint research recognises that the world view of feminist researchers is distinctive and different. There should be a fit, they suggest, between the world view of feminism and the methods adopted for research.

The origins of feminist methodology

Feminist methodology has its roots in feminist theory. Writers such as Millett (1969), Mitchell (1971) and Oakley (1972) and others, particularly in the US and Britain, were the pioneers who helped to direct the focus on women's interests and ideas. Early feminist writers in the professions in Britain include Stanley & Wise (1983) in social work and Webb (1984) in nursing.

A number of major issues emerge in thinking and doing research within a feminist methodological framework:

❑ An initial reaction against positivist research and traditional strategies which are seen as male-dominated and androcentric
❑ An interest in exploring women's perceptions, experiences and feelings. They attempt to make women visible
❑ An emphasis on equality and mutuality which changes the relationship between researcher and researched
❑ The use of **consciousness-raising** as a methodological tool to empower women
❑ The centrality of feminist theory and the aim to add to this through research

Feminist researchers emphasise an alternative social reality and value women's lives and experience. Researchers intend to contribute to the improvement of the lives of women. Feminists are concerned with the importance of women's lives and their position in the social structure. They claim that unequal relations are not only embedded in the structure of society but have taken part in the construction of social relationships.

Feminist thought and methodology

Even before feminism, a disenchantment with natural scientific methods had emerged which led to a critique of *positivism*. Researchers who took the approach of natural science believed that *objectivity* was possible, that to use the scientific method was the best way to examine social reality and would be neutral and objective. Feminists question the notion of value-neutral research and agree with other qualitative researchers who react against the positivist and neo-positivist approach.

Traditional research is also described as male-dominated (Westkott, 1990). Feminist critics of this approach maintain that it is often stripped of its *context* while questions and answers are predefined and controlled by researchers who, whilst claiming objectivity, impose their own subjective framework. Feminists believe that researchers cannot achieve complete objectivity. They can only state their *bias* or assumptions and demonstrate the value bases from which they come; that is, they are reflexive. They criticise the differentiation between the objective and subjective and put an emphasis on the relationships and realities of 'everyday life' through which social structures can be understood.

Women explain their social reality in personal accounts of their lives, and these accounts emerge from their shared experiences. The researcher listens to these accounts and, while interpreting them, gives a faithful picture of the personal histories and biographies of women. Feminist research aims to raise the consciousness of people in general and of the women participants specifically. Consciousness of their reality can guide women to an understanding and helps them to change their lives and empower them. Research makes emotions, personal values and the thoughts of participants legitimate topics of research.

The relationship between researchers and women participants

The *research relationship* follows that of other types of qualitative research but collaboration and equality between the researcher and women participants are stressed even more. Empathy with women may be easier to achieve by female researchers because of their gender (though feminists do not claim that men cannot have empathy, nor that research supports a woman's perspective just because it is done by a woman). The personal experience and values of the researcher become important in feminist research. Feminists often describe and integrate their own feelings while recounting and analysing women's experiences, pains and passions. Sometimes they study women's conditions or problems that they have experienced in their own lives. Feminist qualitative research allows for interactive interviewing where participants can ask questions, both professional and personal.

Researchers try to use consciousness-raising as a tool for narrowing the distance between researchers and participants by generating reciprocity and collaboration. This affects all participants and gives individuals – including researchers – a sense of their identity. Women, so feminists believe, become aware of their position through the research process and relationships; they aim to change their situation and become more powerful.

The researcher herself is a member of a group and can empathise with her informants. That which was assumed to be 'natural', for instance the dominant position of males, can be questioned and even rejected.

The critique of feminist methodology

The critique of feminist research is concerned with issues such as:

❏   The importance of gender and the question of exclusivity
❏   The degree of participant involvement in choice of topic and data analysis
❏   The problem of relativism

One of the critics of feminist methodology is Hammersley (1992) who, nevertheless, acknowledges the importance of research about gender and deplores the neglect of this topic in past research. It is not certain whether researchers who adopt a particular stance and claim superior and unique insight into a group because of their own membership of it are following a sound methodological path. Hammersley sees as relativism the claim by Stanley & Wise (1983) that men and women build different social realities because of their 'different states of consciousness'. The emphasis on the uniqueness of women's experiences ignores the social context which involves more than one gender in his view. One might ask the practical question whether female researchers can ever interview men, or male researchers women. While it would be useful to have a researcher with a similar gender, background, religion or ethnic group as the participant, this is not always practically possible, nor desirable in all cases.

FIELDNOTES

Fieldnotes are records that help the researcher to remember activities, events and people in a setting. The term is used particularly by ethnographers but also by other qualitative researchers. Fieldnotes consist of jottings and writings about experiences in the field and are started as soon as the research begins. Often they are contained in field journals or personal diaries. Fieldnotes encompass raw data from observations and impressions about what researchers find in the field; they include portraits – detailed descriptions – of the informants. They also contain speculations, analytical comments and other thoughts. In short, they are a written account of what goes on in the field: an accurate and detailed description of the setting and context, a faithful report of conversations and a picture of the ongoing actions and interactions without initial evaluation or summary. However, fieldnotes are both **descriptions** and **reflections**. They are written in the *first person* and are read only by the researcher unless he or she decides to share extracts with the readers of the final report.

Fieldnotes can be taken during observations, but informants may feel inhibited if the researcher writes notes while looking and listening. It is important, however, that researchers make fieldnotes during *observations* and as soon as possible after the *interview* because they might not remember clearly what they noticed during fieldwork. The more time goes by the less the researchers remember. Fieldnotes are intended to help them remember what they saw and heard and guide them in their observations. (See also *memoing*.)

It is important to set up an appropriate format for fieldnotes, and they have to be labelled. Researchers should note dates and times before beginning a description of the place and people. It is useful to leave wide margins for further notes or coding of the work. Fieldnotes can also be taped on a tape recorder, but should be transcribed afterwards.

FIELDWORK

Ethnographers and other qualitative researchers use the term fieldwork to describe *data collection* outside laboratories or libraries; researchers conduct their studies in natural settings and work 'in the field' for a period of time ('getting their hands dirty'). Van Maanen (1988) stresses the belief of field-workers in the personal experience of a *culture*. They immerse themselves in the social life of the culture or community, observe its members and interview them while making a written record in *fieldnotes* of details such as patterns of interaction as well as the rules and rituals they observe. Fieldwork informs researchers of events and activities in the setting they study while they are watching people leading their normal, everyday lives. This allows researchers to put these processes into the context of the culture and learn from its members. Researchers are involved in the situation and setting without becoming overinvolved and *going native*.

There is no single way of doing fieldwork. The best studies use a variety of sources for data collection. Fieldwork is not, however, an end in itself, but 'a means to an end' (van Maanen, 1988: 3), that is, the means to produce a picture of the culture under study.

FIRST PERSON

The use of the first person, 'I', can be justified in a qualitative research report as the researcher is the main research tool. The language is not detached and dispassionate because of the researcher's deep involvement and engagement. Geertz (1988) warns against 'author-evacuated' texts. The research is also the result of relationships with others, a 'we'. Shelton-Reed (1997), too, advises writers to speak with 'their own voice'. To speak of 'the author', 'the researcher' or 'the writer' in one's own research report makes the writing lifeless and abnegates the role of the researcher as a research tool (Webb, 1992). Qualitative researchers should be aware, however, that funding agencies often expect the conventional passive form for *research reports*.

FOCUS

The focus of a research project is the main area and interest of the research. The qualitative researcher develops this central idea over time through reading or discussion with experts, through experience or reading. Many studies become progressively more focused on particular issues as the research proceeds. Focused *interviewing*, in particular, centres on the foci of the research. (See also *progressive focusing*.)

FOCUS GROUP

A focus group involves a number of people with common experiences or characteristics whom a researcher (or moderator) interviews for the purpose of eliciting ideas, thoughts and perceptions about a specific topic or certain issues linked to an area of interest. Focus groups are characterised by interaction between the participants from which researchers discover how individuals think and feel about particular issues. The focus group interview is used by researchers in the area of communications, policy, marketing and advertising as well as in social science and the caring professions. The approach to focus group interviews is generally qualitative although it can result in quantitative or multi-method analysis. Focus groups can be combined with individual interviews, observation or other methods of data collection but they do not need to be validated by other methods (Morgan & Krueger, 1993). The findings from the focus group interviews are often used as a basis for action. To give an example of a focus group interview: a doctor interviews small groups of patients who have had heart surgery to find out about their experience in hospital or the rehabilitation process. The processes can be improved through the knowledge gained.

In-depth group interviews have been used by business and market researchers since the 1920s, but the first book on focus groups was written by Merton and his colleagues as a result of working with groups during and shortly after World War II in 1946. Focus groups in the social sciences and health professions have become popular since the growth of qualitative research methods in the last 10 or 20 years.

The sample

The sample is linked closely to the research topic. The topic or the purpose of the focus group generally determines its composition and number. The participants usually have similar roles or experiences; they might share the same speciality, condition or interest, or use the same technical equipment, treatment or procedures. For instance, researchers can interview teachers about the use of video equipment.

The presence of people in a focus group does not mean that they have the same views about the topic area, nor that they come from the same background or organisation. Gender and age as well as social and psychological characteristics of the group members affect the quality and level of interaction and through this the data. The number of focus groups depends on the needs of the researcher and the demands of the topic area. For a single research question the usual number is about three or four, but the actual number depends on the complexity of the research topic.

Group sessions generally last from one to three hours depending on the participants' stamina and time. In market research, participants are paid for their time and effort, but in social research this does not happen because it would coerce, to some extent at least, the informants and squander resources.

Each group contains between three and twelve people. Most books suggest six or seven as the optimum number as it is large enough to provide a variety of perspectives and small enough not to become disorderly or fragmented (Stewart & Shamdasani, 1990). However, experienced researchers find it difficult to work with large groups. Instead their advice is to interview three or four individuals at any one time. Slight over-recruitment for each group is advised in case some individuals are not able to attend. The larger the group, the more problematic the transcription as it can be difficult to distinguish voices. With heterogeneous groups of informants, at least two groups should be conducted with each type so that all informants are interviewed at least twice.

Members of the group, although sharing common experiences, do not have to know each other. Familiarity between participants could lead to dominance of one individual, and the history of the group may inhibit or lead individuals into a particular direction.

The principles of qualitative *data analysis* in focus group interviews are similar to those of other qualitative approaches. A variety of procedures can be adopted (Krueger, 1994).

Conducting focus group interviews

Focus group interviews must be planned carefully. They differ from interviews with individuals in that they explore and stimulate ideas which are produced through **group dynamics** (Greenbaum, 1988). Focus group members respond to the interviewer and each other.

The informants are contacted well before the interviews and reminded a few days before they start. Ethical and access issues are carefully considered. The room must be big enough to contain the participants comfortably, and the tape recorder is placed in an advantageous location, where they can all be heard and recorded. For focus group work, it is even more essential to have a top quality tape recorder than for individual interviews. A circle or semi-circle is the best seating arrangement.

Researchers must identify the agenda, manage time effectively and establish ground rules.

The interviewer

The interviewer becomes the facilitator or moderator in the group discussion. The leadership role of the moderators demands abilities above that of the one-to-one interviewer. A non-directive approach has particular importance in exploratory research where perceptions are examined.

The feelings of the interviewer should not be expressed in the focus group. A special relationship with a specific individual, an affirmative nod at something of which the interviewer approves, or a lack of encouragement for unexpected or unwelcome answers may bias the interviews. Although conflicts of opinion can produce valuable data, the interviewer must defuse personal hostility between members. Gestures and facial expressions have to be controlled to show members of the group that the interviewer is non-judgemental and values the views of all participants.

Strengths and limitations of focus groups

The main strength is the production of data through social interaction and group dynamics. The dynamic interaction stimulates the thoughts of participants (Morgan, 1988) and reminds them of their own feelings about the research topic. Informants build on the answers of others in the group. On responding to each others' comments, informants might generate new and spontaneous ideas which researchers had not thought of before or during the interview. Through interaction informants may remember forgotten feelings and thoughts. All participants, including the interviewer, have the opportunity to ask questions. Kitzinger (1994) also highlights the fact that group interaction might encourage the participants to mention even sensitive topics. Focus groups produce more data in the same space of time; this could make them cheaper and quicker than individual interviews.

There are also some disadvantages. The researcher has less control than in one-to-one interviews. One or two individuals may dominate the discussion and influence the outcome or perhaps even introduce bias as the other members may be merely compliant. A person who is unable to verbalise feelings and thoughts will not make a good informant. Conflict can be destructive but can also generate rich data. In any conflict situation, ethical issues must be carefully considered. As there are certain dangers of group effect and group member control, it is useful to analyse the interviews both at group level and at the level of the individual participants (Carey & Smith, 1994).

Transcription can be much more difficult because people's voices vary and the distance they sit from the microphone influences the clarity of individuals' contributions. Therefore some researchers use video-tapes although this might inhibit the participants.

FOUNDATIONALISM

Foundationalism is a philosophical approach founded on the assumption that knowledge is based on a firm, unquestionable foundation (Phillips, 1993). Rationalism, empiricism and positivism are examples of foundationalism although these schools differ in their ideas about the foundations of knowledge. **Non-foundationalists** believe that knowledge is provisional and tentative. Phillips states that the search for truth has not, however, been given up by non-foundationalists, although all knowledge is thought to be provisional. Most present-day social researchers are non-foundationalists.

FREE LISTING

Free lists are items or ideas that informants generate when being asked about a concept or word that they used while being interviewed or observed. Free listing can define a particular *domain*, or assist in examining social relationships and variations in ideas. Significant items are mentioned more often or appear at the top of the list which informants generate. To be able to use this technique, researchers have to be knowledgeable about the language and *culture* of the informants. Free listing is used in ethnographic studies in particular.

G

GATEKEEPERS

Gatekeepers are individuals or groups who control information and can grant formal or informal *entry* and *access* to the setting and participants; they can impose conditions for access. They may be official, such as the managers of an organisation, or unofficial, namely those persons who might have no formal gatekeeping function but power and influence to grant and deny access. Gatekeepers can be found at any layer of an organisation, at the top level or even at a low level: there is no point in gaining access from management if the rest of the workforce and clients deny or impede it.

Before giving permission for entry, most gatekeepers will wish to be informed about the aims and objectives of the research and its possible outcome and use. They also want to make sure that no risks to themselves, the organisation or its clients exist. If it is likely that the organisation in which the research takes place benefits from it, gatekeepers are more likely to give access.

Researchers expect that gatekeepers do not interfere in the research process (though *ethics committees* can and do). In research carried out with financial and social support from the organisation, there is a danger that gatekeepers have their own expectations and sometimes attempt to manipulate the research – intentionally or unintentionally. This can affect the researchers' direction or reporting of the work, and they might find themselves influenced by these expectations. As gatekeepers are in a position of power over the researcher, resistance might be difficult. For gatekeepers, institutional objectives might take precedence over individual research interest because of the prioritising of resources; for instance, staff time also costs money.

Powerful gatekeepers might see researchers as unsuitable because of gender, youth or behaviour and appearance. They must be convinced that the researcher is trustworthy and able to cope with the study. Friends and acquaintances who are already involved in the researcher's chosen location can sometimes persuade those in power of the ability and trustworthiness of the researcher. If researchers are very young, the gatekeepers might feel that they lack credibility. Managers also deny access when they feel that the setting will be disturbed by the presence of the researcher.

Gatekeepers might prevent or censor publication if they disagree with the researcher's findings or do not wish negative findings to be disclosed to the public. Details about the dissemination of the research should be negotiated with gatekeepers before the research starts so that problems can be avoided.

GENERALISABILITY

Generalisability (or external validity) in research exists when the findings of a study can be applied to other settings and cases or to a whole population, that is, when the findings are true beyond the focus of the work in hand. In traditional research a study was seen as more scientific only if its results were generalisable. The random sampling process ensures that the findings are representative of the population from which the sample was drawn. In qualitative inquiry the question of generalisability is more problematic. Qualitative researchers do not usually claim generalisability of findings because they produce only a slice of the social situation rather than the whole; indeed they state that the concept of generalisability might be irrelevant if they examine a single case or a unique phenomenon. Strauss & Corbin (1990) speak of **representativeness of *concepts*** and **applicability of *theory***. Researchers generalise because they have gained knowledge of the concepts, instances and conditions about the phenomenon under study. Morse (1994) claims that theory contributes to the 'greater body of knowledge' when it is 'recontextualised' into a variety of settings; therefore she uses the phrase '**theory-based generalisation**'. It involves the application of theoretical concepts found in one situation to other settings and conditions. If the theory developed from the original *data analysis* can be verified in other sites and situations, the theoretical ideas are generalisable. (There has been a change in terminology in much qualitative research. See *validity*.)

In any case, the purpose of qualitative research is to uncover the **essence** of a phenomenon, not to generalise from a single case or a small number of cases. In this respect qualitative research has **specificity**; some researchers even claim that large sample size, far from being useful, prevents examination of meaning and context (Banister *et al.*, 1994). Payne & Cuff (1982), however, argue that generalisations from a few cases are possible; just as a small group of statements can establish generalisations about an entire language, so individual cases can do the same for a subculture.

Researchers gain knowledge of many concepts and instances about the phenomenon examined which they can then transfer to other situations. Theories which are learnt from a small number of cases can often be transferred to a larger number. Therefore they have theory-based generality. Qualitative researchers often – if not always – produce a description and analysis of reality that is 'typical' for a particular setting by taking into account the conditions and the context under which the phenomena occur. **Typicality** is achieved when experiences and perceptions of a specific sample are 'typical' of the phenomenon under study and relate to the theoretical ideas which have emerged. It is useful, even in qualitative research, to demonstrate relationships that go beyond the immediate situation.

Generalisations can be made if they are supported by evidence from a number of other sources, which happens, for instance, if multi-site research is carried out; qualitative researchers also use the relevant research literature as data which are added to a study as additional findings. They take into account the number of studies focusing on similar topics, populations and methods; through this, generalisation and typicality can be achieved. Each piece of research contributes to the whole and the broader scheme. Individual cases point to a larger picture.

'GOING NATIVE'

Researchers 'go native' when they submerge themselves in the *culture* they research and become part of it. The term originated in *anthropology* but is now used in other types of *qualitative research*. When they 'go native', researchers adopt the values and perspectives of the people they study, and identify with them so much that they are unable to sustain their previous identity as researchers. This prevents them from maintaining their research roles and eliminates any element of objectivity. It happens occasionally in participant observation projects.

Immersion in the culture under study is important because it helps researchers learn about it. They become less visible, and this lessens the observer effect (see *reactivity*) which 'strangers' to the setting might generate. On the one hand, the researchers have to involve and immerse themselves in the culture; on the other, there is the danger that they identify too closely with the people they study and cannot maintain their researcher roles. 'Going native' also means that they might not maintain their critical stance towards the issues under investigation.

GROUNDED THEORY

Grounded theory (GT) is an approach to *data collection* and *data analysis* initially developed by Barney Glaser and Anselm Strauss in the 1960s. It aims to develop theory from the data collected by the researcher. It has its origins in sociology, particularly *symbolic interactionism*. These two sociologists advanced qualitative approaches from their early, less systematic tradition. Charmaz (1995) asserts that Glaser and Strauss developed *qualitative research* by the following means:

(1)   They closed the arbitrary gap between *theory* and research.
(2)   They stated that qualitative research could stand on its own and does not have to be merely an exploratory tool for a quantitative study.
(3)   Through their work, qualitative research was made more rigorous and systematic.
(4)   Data collection and data analysis became an interactive process.
(5)   They also asserted that GT was not merely description but con-ceptualisation; researchers had to generate and develop theory.

Glaser (1992) claims that grounded theory methods are not specific to a particular discipline or type of data collection. GT can be used in any field of study in an orderly and systematic way, be it psychology, health or business studies, and for any type of material, such as interview transcripts, observations or documents and diaries. Researchers use grounded theory to investigate interactions, behaviours and experiences as well as individuals' perceptions and thoughts about them. Grounded theory stresses the importance of *context* in which people function and the roles they adopt in interaction.

Strauss (1987) maintained that it is not a particular technique but 'a style of doing qualitative analysis' with distinct characteristics. Grounded theory is more structured than other forms of qualitative research, although it uses similar approaches to data collection and analysis. It is sometimes suggested that qualitative methods produce descriptive studies; Strauss & Corbin (1990) firmly deny this. They state that a grounded theory must not just be descriptive but should also have explanatory power.

Glaser and Strauss worked together on research about health professionals' interaction with dying patients and through this generated two books (Glaser & Strauss, 1965, 1968) which have become exemplars for grounded theory. From research and teaching the classic text emerged, *The Discovery of Grounded Theory* (Glaser & Strauss, 1967). Four other books on grounded theory followed: *Field Research: Strategies for a Natural Sociology* (Schatzman & Strauss, 1973), *Theoretical Sensitivity* (Glaser, 1978), *Qualitative Analysis for Social Scientists* (Strauss, 1987), and *The Basics of Qualitative Research* (Strauss & Corbin, 1990). The last – in which Strauss co-authors with a nurse researcher – is by far the clearest and most practically useful book on grounded theory as it describes an approach that has been tried and clarified over time. The book has been strongly criticised by Glaser (1992) who attempts to refute Strauss and Corbin's text. He claims, *inter alia*, that these authors distort the main ideas of GT by forcing the data and making the research verificational. He calls the 1990 approach 'conceptual description' rather than grounded theory. Melia (1996) enters the debate by sympathising with Glaser. However, although she calls the Strauss and Corbin book somewhat 'formulaic', she still recognises it as a description of GT. Ultimately she sees the debate as an 'academic difference of opinion'. There now seem to be Glaserian and Straussian versions of GT (Stern, 1994; Melia, 1996), with different schools and loyalties.

The aims of grounded theory

The main aim of grounded theory is the **generation of theory from the data**, although existing theories can be modified or extended through this approach. It emphasises the development of ideas from the data like other qualitative methods but goes further than these. Grounded theory researchers start with an area of interest, collect the data and allow the relevant ideas to develop.

Rigid preconceived ideas prevent development of the research; imposing a framework might block the awareness of major concepts that emerge from the data. Grounded theory is especially useful in situations where little is known about a particular topic or problem area, or where a new and exciting outlook is needed in familiar settings.

The grounded theory style of research uses ***constant comparison***. The researcher compares each section of the data with every other part throughout the study for similarities, differences and connections. Included in this process are the *themes* and *categories* identified in the literature. All the data are coded and categorised, and from this process major *concepts* and *constructs* are formed. The researcher takes up a search for major themes which link ideas to find a *storyline* for the study.

The approach is initially **inductive**. It also uses **deductive** processes. (See *induction* and *deduction*.) Grounded theory does not start with a hypothesis. After collecting the initial data, however, relationships are established and provisional hypotheses or propositions conceived (a provisional hypothesis or proposition in qualitative research is sometimes called a 'working hypothesis'). These are checked out against further data. (See *hypothesis*.)

Grounded theorists accept their role as interpreters of the data and do not stop at merely reporting them. Researchers search for relationships between concepts and find patterns and links from which they develop theories. Grounded theorists are systematic and detailed in their approach to the data.

Features of grounded theory

Researchers must have *theoretical sensitivity*, which means that they develop insight and awareness of relevant and significant ideas while collecting and analysing the data. Sensitivity is built up over time, from reading and experience. It guides the researcher to examine the data from all sides rather than staying fixed on the obvious. There are a variety of sources for *theoretical sensitivity*. Professional experience can be one source of awareness, and personal experiences, too, can help make the researcher sensitive. The literature too, sensitises in the sense that documents, research studies or autobiographies create awareness in the researcher of relevant and significant elements in the data. When researchers manage the data, theoretical sensitivity develops gradually because they think about emerging ideas, ask further questions and see these ideas as provisional until they have been examined over time, linked back to the data and, finally, confirmed by the data.

Sampling guided by ideas which have significance for the emerging theory is called **theoretical sampling**. The difference between theoretical and other types of sampling concerns time and continuance. Unlike other sampling which is planned beforehand, theoretical sampling in grounded theory continues throughout the study and is not planned in detail before the study starts. Theoretical sampling, though originating in grounded theory, is also often used in other types of qualitative analysis. Finch & Mason (1990: 28) explain theoretical sampling: 'Essentially theoretical sampling means selecting a study population on theoretical rather than, say, statistical grounds.'

At the start of the project researchers make initial sampling decisions. They choose a setting and particular participants able to give information on the topic under study. Once the research has started and initial data have been analysed, new concepts arise, and events and people are chosen for further illumination of the problem. Researchers then set out to sample different situations, individuals or a variety of settings, and focus on new ideas to extend the emerging theories. The selection of participants, settings, events or documents is a function of developing theories. Theoretical sampling continues until the point of *saturation*. Researchers often believe that saturation has taken place when a concept is mentioned frequently and described in similar ways by a number of people, or when the same ideas arise repeatedly. This does not necessarily mean that saturation has occurred. It has been obtained when the theory fully explains variations in the data. Saturation is achieved at a different stage in each research project and cannot be predicted.

Data collection

Data collection takes place through observations in the field, interviews of participants, and through reading diaries and other documents such as letters or even newspapers. Researchers use interviews and observations more often than other data sources, and they supplement these through literature searches. Indeed, the literature becomes part of the data that are analysed. Everything, even experiences of researchers, can become sources of data. Glaser & Strauss (1967) advise that the researchers be flexible, approach the study with an open mind and avoid assumptions before the study starts.

Data collection and analysis are linked from the beginning of the research and interact continuously. The analysis starts after the first few steps in the data collection have been taken; the emerging ideas guide the analysis. The gathering of data does not finish until the end of the research because ideas, concepts and new questions continually arise which guide the researcher to new data sources. Researchers collect data from initial interviews or observations and take their cues from the first emerging ideas to develop further interviews and observations. This means that the collection of data becomes more focused and specific as the process develops (see *progressive focusing*).

While observing and interviewing, the investigator writes **memos** (see *memoing*) throughout the project from the beginning of the data collection. Certain occurrences in the setting or ideas from the participants that seem of vital interest are recorded either during or immediately after data collection. They remind the researcher of the events, actions and interactions and trigger thinking processes.

Data analysis

The process of *data analysis* goes on throughout the research from the first interview and observation to the last. Analysis initially consists of **coding** and **categorising**. From the start of the study, analysts code the data. *Coding* in grounded theory is the process by which concepts or themes are identified and named during the analysis. Data are transformed and reduced to build categories. Through the emergence of major categories, *theory* can evolve.

There are three steps in the coding process. The first is concerned with open coding which starts as soon as the researcher receives the data and examines them. **Open coding** is the process of breaking down and conceptualising the data. Each separate idea in the data is given a label. Similar ideas are named with the same label.

Sometimes these codes consist of words and phrases used by the participants themselves to describe a phenomenon. They are called '**in vivo codes**'. These can give life and interest to the study and can be immediately recognised as reflecting the reality of the participants. An in vivo code might be the expression 'thrown in at the deep end' for a study of socialisation, for instance. The participants themselves use this expression.

In grounded theory, all the data are coded, generally line by line, or paragraph by paragraph, in interviews and fieldnotes. Initial codes tend to be provisional and are modified or transformed over the period of analysis. At the beginning of a project or a study, line-by-line analysis is important, although it may be a long drawn-out process for analysts. Codes are based directly on the data so that the researcher avoids preconceived ideas.

At the start a great number of labels are used. After initial coding, analysts condense (or collapse) codes into groups of concepts with similar traits. These are called **categories**. Categories tend to be more abstract than initial codes and are generally formulated by the investigator who always refers back to the data. The main features (properties) and dimensions of these categories are identified. Initially it is advised to code line by line. When researchers have become familiar with the data they might code by paragraphs or extract the significant themes.

The researchers go on to **axial coding** where they reassemble the data broken down through open coding. Categories are grouped together in a new form to build major categories. Researchers label these. Occasionally they use labels that others have discovered before them and that are found in the literature.

The process starts with open coding and then continues to axial coding. After this it alternates between the two.

Although there is no initial hypothesis in grounded theory, during the course of the research working hypotheses or propositions are generated. These must be based in and indicated by the data. The process of checking the working hypotheses goes on throughout the research. This includes the search for deviant or negative cases which do not support a particular *proposition*. When these are found, the researcher must modify the hypothesis or find reasons why it is not applicable in this particular instance.

The process of coding and categorising only stops when

❏ no new information on a category can be found in spite of the attempt to collect more data from a variety of sources
❏ the category has been described with all its properties, variations and processes
❏ links between categories are firmly established (Corbin & Strauss, 1990)

The third step for the researcher is **selective coding** which is coding for the main phenomenon, the **core category** (also called the core variable), the major category that in grounded theory links all others. Like a thread the category should be integrated and provide the story line. The linking of all categories around a core is called selective coding. This means that the researcher uncovers the essence of the study and integrates all the elements of the emergent theory. Included in the core category are the ideas that are most significant to the participants.

Coding and categorising involve **constant comparison**. Initial interviews are analysed, and codes and concepts developed. By comparing concepts and subcategories, researchers are able to group them into major categories and label them. When they code and categorise incoming data, they compare new categories with those that have already been established. Thus, incoming data are checked for their 'fit' with existing categories. Each incident of a category is compared with every other incident for similarities and differences. The comparison involves the literature. Constant comparison is useful for finding the properties and dimensions of categories. It assists in looking at concepts critically as each concept is illuminated by the new, incoming data.

Generation of theory

To be credible the theory must have 'explanatory power', linkages between categories and specificity. Categories are connected with each other and tightly linked to the data. Researchers do not just describe static situations but take into account processes in the setting under study. Glaser & Strauss (1967) state that two types of theory are produced: substantive and formal theory. **Substantive theory** emerges from a study of just one particular context – for instance a business firm, a hospital ward, or a classroom: hence this type of theory is very useful for researchers in the professions. It has specificity and applies to the setting and situation studied; this means that it is limited. **Formal theory** is generated from many different situations and settings, is conceptual and has higher generality. One can give an example of the two types of theory. The idea that there are stages through which dying patients in hospital proceed is substantive theory. When this is linked to the existence of a 'status passage' which can be applied to many situations where people pass through stages, it becomes formal theory. The latter type of theory has general applicability. It holds true not just for the setting of the specific study but also for other settings and situations. In a small student project, it would be difficult to produce a formal theory with wide applications, but substantive theories can also be important and have general implications.

Glaser & Strauss (1967) maintain that grounded theory is superior to grand theory exemplified by the sociologist Talcott Parsons and the middle range theory of Robert Merton. As these latter theories are not rooted in research, they are merely speculative.

The place of the literature

The literature becomes a source for data. When categories have been found, researchers trawl the literature for confirmation or refutation of these categories. They try to discover what other researchers have found, and whether there are any links to existing theories. The literature becomes part of the data. Although there is an initial literature review to demonstrate the gap in knowledge, the rest of the literature becomes integrated into the final write-up of the study. (See Strauss & Corbin, 1990.)

Memoing takes place throughout the study. Memos are comments and explanations about the codes and categories written by researchers during the collection and analysis of data. Memos trace patterns in the data and contribute to the analysis.

Problems and pitfalls

Occasional problems of GT can be identified. Becker (1993) argues that some of the studies with this approach seem too descriptive. Researchers produce good stories including categories or types but often neglect the underlying social processes and abstract concepts. She stresses the need for qualitative researchers to give explanations, not just descriptions, and this is important particularly in GT. Strauss & Corbin (1990) emphasise the difference between description and conceptualisation. It is not enough to describe the perspectives of the participant to develop a truly 'grounded' theory.

The term 'emerging categories' or 'emerging theory' is criticised by Stern (1994) who maintains that these do not simply 'emerge' as if arising by magic. They have to be worked for and 'pulled' from the data.

Another problem concerns theoretical sampling. Often researchers use selective (or purposive) sampling procedures on which they decide before data collection. For grounded theory research this does not suffice. Theoretical sampling is necessary because of the inductive–deductive nature of the research. Induction is linked to emerging theories which researchers try to advance through theoretical sampling.

H

HERMENEUTICS

Hermeneutics is a way of interpreting human behaviour; it is thus an area in interpretive *methodology*. The Greek god Hermes, 'the messenger', who interpreted messages from Zeus to human beings, gave his name to hermeneutics. Originally developed as a term for the interpretation of biblical texts after the reformation, hermeneutics focuses on the interpretation of the experience shared by human beings and on empathetic understanding. It is believed that human consciousness and interpretation construct reality, and therefore texts can be interpreted in many different ways.

In social science the concept was developed by Dilthey (1833–1911), the German philosopher. Hermeneutic phenomenologists (such as Heidegger and Ricoeur) show that human actions appear to the observer as a written text appears to the reader. The best known modern proponents of hermeneutics are Gadamer and Habermas. Gadamer (1960) asserts that the interpreters of the text construct or reconstruct history. He claims that while readers interpret a text they cannot separate themselves from its meaning. This means that there is interaction between the text and the interpreter of the text.

Gadamer explains the 'hermeneutic circle'. A hermeneutic circle means that a text is understood by reference to the *context* in which it was generated; the text in turn produces an understanding of the originator and context. Parts of the text are understood by reference to the whole, and the whole is understood in terms of its parts. Scott (1990) explains that the circle is entered by the researcher whose dialogue with the text becomes part of the circle. Habermas (1972, 1974), a German social theorist and philosopher, points out the importance of meaningful understanding and human communication in hermeneutic inquiry. He believes that human beings are so embedded in the world that they can never wholly bracket or suspend their prejudices and that all knowledge involves interests and traditions.

As van Manen (1990) suggests, lived experience is grasped through language which he calls 'the human science text', and it is interpreted. Researchers examine human actions like texts in which they find underlying meanings. Actions provide access to the meaning context. Usher & Bryant (1989) show that, according to Gadamer, hermeneutic understanding takes a central role in human practice.

Researchers using hermeneutic *phenomenology* gather *data* from language, texts and actions. They have to return to the data frequently, and ask the *participants* what the data mean to them. Every time they return to the participants' world, they gain more understanding and knowledge about it and so increase their understanding. Sometimes meanings have to be revised.

The researcher goes beyond the accounts of the participant. The participant as the original creator of the data, and the researcher as their interpreter, together generate the data; the meanings of the participant and the meanings of the researcher are integrated with each other. Researchers attempt to gain an understanding of the context which gives meaning to the data.

HEURISTIC DEVICE

A heuristic device is a conceptualisation that assists in understanding and guides researchers towards discovery (the Greek *heuriskein* means 'to discover'). Weber's *ideal type* is a heuristic device (Williams & May, 1996).

HEURISTIC RESEARCH

Heuristic research explores the process of discovering meaning in the experience of individuals. It enables the development of strategies for further exploration. Moustakas (1990) is the main user of this term. Heuristic research can be considered a form of phenomenological research. (See *phenomenology*.)

HISTORICAL RESEARCH

Historical research is an investigation of history. Most historical research is both qualitative and quantitative. It focuses on historical documents such as letters, diaries or writing by historians as well as on records such as parish or town hall records. Artefacts, reports of eyewitnesses or films are also examined for inquiries into the recent past. A study of hospitals in the nineteenth century, for instance, could include contemporary drawings or letters from patients or nurses and documents from the hospitals. All these become data. Qualitative researchers analyse the data in a similar way as they would other types of research. In historical research, the context is of particular importance. (See also *documentary sources*.)

HYPOTHESIS

A hypothesis is a proposition or untested theory about relationships between *concepts*. It is presented for empirical testing or assessment, for verification or falsification. For instance: 'young people do not comply with doctors' suggestions' might be a hypothesis that could be tested.

In general, qualitative research does not start with a hypothesis because it is initially inductive (see *induction*) but generates and develops working hypotheses or propositions and attempts to examine whether they fit the data. (In *grounded theory* these are initially the relationships between *categories* and their properties.) Researchers develop initial explanations and definitions of a phenomenon and compare them with the incoming *data*. If these contradict or do not fit the earlier ideas, researchers reformulate the working hypothesis.

Silverman (1993: 28) stresses that hypothesis testing is 'not only practical but often desirable'. One could claim this also for the working hypotheses or propositions in qualitative research where hypotheses may be developed and tested during the course of qualitative analysis as *theory* is generated.

I

ICONIC STATEMENT

An iconic statement (Rubin & Rubin, 1995) is a summary of the participants' interpretations of a significant aspect of their world or a brisk statement about an important problem or its solution. Consider these statements made by a social work teacher: 'When I first came to university, I had no idea about teaching, I was thrown in at the deep end. I used those teachers as role models whom I had met during my own school career.'

IDEAL TYPE

An ideal type is a *construct* that is a description of a phenomenon in its abstract form. Max Weber (1864–1920) used and developed this term. Ideal types do not exist in their pure form. An example: sociologists often use the constructs 'working class' and 'middle class' and give the two groups particular characteristics. These conceptualisations do not exist in empirical reality but are the end of a continuum into which groups of people fit.

The ideal type can assist researchers to compare and classify phenomena. For instance, the researcher might construct an active and a passive model of patient behaviour. He or she can then compare reality in the doctor–patient interaction with this ideal type. This construct may lead to working propositions.

IDEALISM

Idealism, in contrast to *realism*, is an approach that claims that the social world is a created and interpreted world and that descriptions of it cannot accurately reflect reality. People are both subject and object of study, so the research can never be objective or divorced from its context.

IDENTIFIER

This is the pseudonym, letter or number by which a *participant* in the research process can be identified. For reasons of anonymity and other ethical considerations, this is not a real name. Researchers often use an identifier when giving direct *quotes* to demonstrate that the quotes do not come solely from one or two participants but indicate overall patterns (taking care that the real identity of the participants stays hidden).

IDIOGRAPHIC

The term derives from the Greek, and means 'describing individual, unique persons or events'. Idiographic methods are those in which the individual case has primacy and where lawlike generalities are not sought. These methods focus, according to Windelband, Dilthey and Weber, on ideas about knowledge in the social (human or cultural) sciences rather than in the natural sciences with their *nomothetic* methods. Max Weber (1864–1920), one of the great sociological writers, tried to establish a *methodology* in social science (Geisteswissenschaft), distinguishing it from natural science (Naturwissenschaft). These ideas had their origin in nineteenth century Germany in the philosophical debate about these sciences; the naturalists maintained that the same methodology could be applied in both natural and social sciences while others, such as Dilthey, demanded different methods. This debate was called 'Methodenstreit', that is, conflict about methods.

INDUCTION

Inductive reasoning means going from the specific to the general, that is, starting with the observation or study of a number of individual cases or incidents and establishing generalities that link them to each other. Researchers collect data (without making prior assumptions), analyse the data and generate theories. Bacon (1561–1626), who developed early ideas on induction, argued for the inclusion of *negative cases* now recognised as important for the prevention of *premature closure* in qualitative research. Most qualitative research starts with inductive strategies, although it becomes deductive in approaches where researchers produce working propositions. (See *hypothesis*.)

INFORMED CONSENT

Informed consent is one of the ethical and legal stipulations for research and should always be obtained by the researcher. The participants must be informed about the details of the research and their place in it. In pre-interview contact, the researchers should give their own details and the purpose of their inquiry.

The interviewer or observer details include the following:

(1)   The name, status and address of the interviewer and his or her agency or organisation.
(2)   The aim of the research and its eventual or potential use.
(3)   The reason why the individual was chosen to participate.
(4)   The risk (if there is one) to the informant.
(5)   The information that the participants can withdraw at any time from the research if they wish to do so.
(6)   The statement that the participant's treatment or management will not be affected by the research.

In a qualitative study it is difficult to give all information because detailed ideas emerge and are not fully formed at the beginning of the research. The guarantee of the participant's **right to withdraw** is therefore important. (See also *ethics*.)

INQUIRY AUDIT

The inquiry audit is a systematic evaluation process of research to establish its quality (Schwandt & Halpern, 1988). The term 'audit' originates in business where financial auditors examine the evidence and make judgements about the procedures and quality of an organisation. In a qualitative inquiry audit the researchers' peers review the study, applying certain criteria to evaluate it and checking its **trustworthiness** and authenticity. The inquiry audit is necessary to assure the research's readers and *audience* of its trustworthiness. The researcher therefore has to supply an ***audit trail***. This provides evidence in the form of data and documents such as excerpts from *fieldnotes*, transcripts, research diaries, etc. which the researcher's peers, the 'auditors' of the research, can follow.

INTERPRETIVISM

Interpretivism or the interpretive (interpretative or interpretivist) approach is a direction in social science that focuses on human beings and their way of interpreting and making sense of reality. The interpretive model has its roots in philosophy and the human sciences, particularly in history and anthropology. Researchers should approach participants not as individual entities who exist in a vacuum but within the whole context of their lives. Social scientists who focus on this model believe that understanding human experiences is as important as the ideas of the positivist paradigm which emphasises explanation, prediction and control. This interpretive model has a long history and includes nineteenth century historians, Weberian sociology and approaches such as *symbolic interactionism* and *ethnomethodology*. Philosophers such as Dilthey (1833–1911) considered that the social sciences should not imitate the natural sciences but have their own way of researching.

The interpretivist paradigm can be linked to Weber's *Verstehen* approach. Weber, too, was well aware of the two paradigms in the nineteenth century. He believed that social scientists should be concerned with the interpretive understanding of human beings. Weber argued that 'understanding' in the social sciences is inherently different from 'explanation' in the natural sciences. He differentiates between the *nomothetic*, rule-governed methods of the latter and *idiographic* methods focusing on individual cases and not linked to the general laws of nature but to the actions of human beings. Weber believed that numerically measured probability is quantitative only and wanted to stress that social science concerns itself with the qualitative. We should treat the people we study, he advised, 'as if they were human beings' and try to gain access to their experiences and perceptions by listening to them and observing them.

Most qualitative research has its origin in the interpretive perspective. Throughout the research, investigators in qualitative inquiry turn to the human participants for guidance, control and direction. Interpretive researchers also claim that the experiences of people are essentially context-bound and not free from time, location or the mind of the human *actor*. Researchers must understand the socially constructed nature of the social world and realise that values and interests become part of the research process. Researchers are not divorced from the phenomenon under study. Language itself is context-bound and depends on the researchers' and informants' values and social location. This means *reflexivity* on their part; they must take into account their own position in the setting as they are the main research tool.

INTERSUBJECTIVITY

This term originated with Husserl (1859–1938) who wished to know about the processes by which human beings share the world with each other. Weber's notion of *Verstehen* – empathetic understanding – is similar to this. Schütz (1967) also developed the term. He claimed that human beings believe in reciprocity of perspectives that are accessible to the members of their culture. In qualitative research, understanding means that the members of a culture or society share the meanings they give to their actions and perceptions. Inter-subjectivity may give rise to commonalities in the *data* which produce *categories* and *constructs*.

INTERVIEW

The qualitative **in-depth interview** has become a favoured strategy of *data collection* in qualitative research and produces 'rich' data. A variety of terms are used for qualitative interviewing, for instance: depth interviewing, intensive interviewing, non-directive interviewing, conversational interviewing, narrative interviewing, and biographical interviewing (Weiss, 1994). The qualitative interview is a 'conversation with a purpose' in which the interviewer aims to obtain the perspectives, feelings and perceptions from the *participant(s)* in the research. It can be formal or informal. **Informal interviews** are conversations where an observer might ask about the observed activities. **Formal interviews** are more likely to be set up in advance and tape-recorded. There could be individual, one-to-one interviews or *focus-group* interviews. Researchers use interviews as the main mode of data collection or parallel to other types of data gathering. Often they take place when researchers wish to explore issues which have become obvious in observations. The interview makes it possible for the informant to take a perspective on the past or discuss the future. This is its advantage over *observation*.

Qualitative interviews differ in their degree of structure. Researchers use

❑ unstructured, non-standardised interviews
❑ semi-structured interviews

The **unstructured interview** begins with a broad, open-ended question within the topic area, such as 'Tell me about . . .' or 'What is your experience of . . .', or 'What is your view on . . .'. The researcher uses an *aide mémoire* with key points to remind the researcher of the particular areas of interest in the research. In this type of interview the interviewer has minimal control and follows up the ideas of the participants while they tell their story. Unstructured interviews are useful when little is known about the area of study. A *life history* or *narrative* is also elicited through unstructured interviewing. The unstructured interview generates the richest data, but it also has the highest '*dross rate*' (the amount of material of no particular use for the researcher's study), especially with an inexperienced interviewer. **Prompts**, that are short questions, can be used to develop ideas. For instance, the researcher asks, 'Can you tell me more about this?', 'What do you mean?', 'Could you develop this?', etc. In life histories or narratives there is not much *questioning*. Questions can be reformulated throughout the interview.

The **semi-structured interview** has a more specific research agenda and is more focused (it is also called the focused interview), but the informants in this type of interview, too, describe the situation in their own words and in their own time. Although researchers do not ask the questions in the same way and form of each participant, they can ensure through the tighter structure of semi-structured interviews that they collect all important information about the research topic while still giving informants the opportunity to report on their own thoughts and feelings.

The questions are contained in an **interview guide** (not schedule as in quantitative research!) with a focus on the issues to be covered. This is particularly relevant in later interviews where researchers start to develop theory. The dross rate is lower than in unstructured interviews.

The sequencing of questions depends on the process of the interview and the answers of each individual, and therefore it is not the same for each participant. Researchers can develop questions and decide which issues to pursue. Interviews may become more guided through *progressive focusing*, particularly when researchers use *grounded theory*, but they should take care not to control the answers and instead to be guided by the informants' ideas and thoughts.

In qualitative inquiry it is possible to re-examine the issues, follow emerging ideas and interview for a second or third time. Seidmann (1991) sees three interviews as the optimum number, but these would be difficult to carry out in the short timespan available to some researchers. Many qualitative researchers use one-off interviews. The sequencing of questions is not the same for every participant as it depends on the process of the interview and the answers of each individual. However, the interview guide ensures that the researcher collects similar types of data from all informants. In this way, the interviewer can save time. Researchers can develop questions and decide for themselves which issues to pursue.

Researchers have to be aware of **interviewer bias**. The term *bias* is not often used in qualitative research. Nevertheless, as the most important instrument in qualitative research, the researcher can influence the study both negatively or positively depending on a number of factors which can interfere. These may be gender, ethnicity or any other group membership of the researchers as well as their stance and assumptions. Lack of rapport or over-rapport between interviewer and informant could also affect the outcome of a study. Biases and assumptions should be stated. (The *subjectivity* of the researcher can, however, become a resource.)

The duration of the qualitative interview differs from about 45 minutes to an hour and a half or more, depending on the time and stamina of the participants (one of my colleagues carried out three-hour interviews because the participants wished to talk). An oral history or *life history* interview generally takes much longer. This type of interview demands prolonged engagement between interviewer and informant.

INTRODUCTION

The introduction to a research report is the justification of a study which sets the scene and describes the setting. It consists of the background and context of the research as well as the **aim** of the project. In qualitative research the aim can be placed at the beginning or end of the introduction. Generally the statement of the study's aim should not contain more than a maximum of 25 words to maintain clarity and simplicity. Writers explain in the introduction why they have become interested in the *research question*, how their project relates to the general topic area, and what gap in knowledge they might fill by the research; therefore the initial *literature review* generally becomes part of the introduction. In qualitative research the writers can include their own experiences as a reason for the research.

ITERATION

Iteration in qualitative research means the return to the sources of the emerging *concepts* in order to examine whether these are truly grounded in the *data*. This process is repeated and becomes circular where there is continuous movement between data and ideas (Coffey & Atkinson, 1996). Qualitative researchers also return to questions they have asked previously, and they repeat these questions and ask them in different ways. This again is part of the iterative process. Most *qualitative research* is iterative. Geertz (1976) calls this movement between different elements of the study 'tacking' (a term originating in the language of sailors).

K

KEY INFORMANT

Key informants are persons who have special knowledge about the history and *culture* of a group, about interaction processes in it and cultural rules, rituals and language. As active *participants* in the setting, they have spent more time and have more experience of the setting than other informants. Key informants tell the researcher about the setting. They are 'guides to insider understandings' (Lofland & Lofland, 1995).

The term has its origin in *anthropology*. Key informants help the researcher to become accepted in the culture and subculture. Researchers can validate their own ideas or perceptions with those of key informants by going back to them at the end of the study and asking them to check the script and interpretation. In qualitative research this is called *member check*.

The bond between researcher and key informant strengthens when the two spend time with each other. Through informal conversations, researchers can learn about the customs and conduct of the group they study because key informants have access to areas which researchers cannot reach because they live in a different time and different location. Key informants share their special knowledge to fill gaps in the researcher's knowledge; they are 'culturally competent' people. Spradley (1979) advises ethnographers to elicit the *tacit knowledge* of cultural members, the concepts and assumptions they have and of which they are often unaware. Researchers must guard against key informants' prior assumptions (Fetterman, 1989). If they are highly knowledgeable, they might impose their own ideas on the study and the researcher, or they might unconsciously mislead. The researcher must therefore try to compare informant tales with the observed reality. There might be the additional danger that key actors might only tell what researchers wish to hear. However, the lengthy contact of interviewer and informants helps to overcome this. It is better to have a number of key informants rather than just one.

L

LIFE HISTORY

A life history is a form of *narrative*. Life histories differ from narratives by being structured in chronological sequence covering a long period of time. They are retrospective reports by individuals about their own lives and development, sometimes including work or illness careers. Not only do life histories help researchers to understand the personal lives of people within a *culture*; they may also teach researchers about this culture and its values and norms. What is more important, researchers might come to understand the reasons for people's beliefs and behaviour. Goodson (1992) argues that there is a difference between life histories and life stories, seeing life history as a story that individuals tell, embedded in its historical context, whereas life stories are stories of participants' lives which are not necessarily given in chronological order.

LIMITATION

The limitations of the design and methods of a project are its restrictions and shortcomings. These are weaknesses over which the researcher has no control. They should be stated openly at the same time as the researcher explains the advantages and strengths of the design (in commercial research this is, of course, not always advisable). The readers can then judge for themselves whether researchers allow for, or overcome, the limitations of the research. For instance, one of the limitations of qualitative research is its lack of representativeness. Researchers have to explain that they rarely aim at this as generalisability is not usually an issue in qualitative research. (See also *delimitation* and *generalisability*.)

LITERATURE REVIEW

The literature review is an overview of the literature in the general topic area of the research. It has a different place in qualitative studies from the review in quantitative research. The literature review in the former is an **initial literature review**.

Of course, a qualitative literature review shows some of the relevant research that has been done in the same field or topic area, and in this respect is similar to other research proposals and reports. The researchers trawl the relevant and related literature, summarise the main ideas from these studies as well as some of the problems and contradictions found, and show how they relate to the proposed project. However, it is not necessary in qualitative reports to review every piece of known research in the field nor to give a critical review of all the literature from the very beginning of the project. The initial literature review should consist of the main pertinent studies including classic and most recent research, as well as the methodological approaches and procedures used for them. Gaps in current knowledge become apparent at this point. The researcher wants to fill these, thereby justifying the research and presenting a coherent argument for it. At this stage, the *research question* is linked to the literature.

By the end of the introductory section, the reader should be in no doubt that a qualitative study, in the form described by the researcher, is most appropriate to meet the research aim.

M

MAPPING

Researchers get involved in the setting, look at the site, and talk and listen to possible *participants*. While examining the main features of the situation and the actions and beliefs of cultural members, they map out the territory. This happens in the initial stages of a project. Through this they find out about the type of possible informant.

MATRIX

A matrix is a visual display of a typology or cross-classification in diagrammatic form. It consists of rows and columns (Miles & Huberman, 1994). In *qualitative research*, matrices generally contain words that present the research findings. A matrix helps the researcher to organise the findings and makes them easily and quickly available to readers so that they can make sense of the data. The simplest matrix is one with two dimensions in rows and columns, but many different forms are possible (Robson, 1993). Matrices generally do not present all the *data*. This means that only the most important dimensions are shown. Explicit rules and detailed records for inclusion exist.

MEANING

Human beings give meaning to their actions and interaction with others. They make sense of their experiences, and qualitative researchers wish to find out how this is done. Informants can reconstruct the past and speculate about its influence on the present. In *interviews*, diaries and *narratives*, they interpret events and experience. The informants' meaning-making processes become the focus of the researcher.

MEMBER CHECK

Member check (sometimes called 'respondent or participant validation') is a term used by Lincoln & Guba (1985). Researchers verify their findings through member check, returning to the *participants* for their response to the findings and interpretations. The participants in a setting have the opportunity to comment and indicate whether they recognise their own experiences from these and/or to give additional information. A member check provides a type of *triangulation* (Hoffart, 1991). This means researchers checking the interpretation of data by asking informants about them, either formally or informally. They show the participants the whole of the *transcript* or a summary. It is better to show a summary or the interpretation itself because reading through the whole transcript takes up too much time. Also, participants might feel overburdened, particularly if they are very young or very old.

The member check may be problematic for a number of reasons.

❑ It is difficult for participants to be objective about the interpretations made by the researcher, and they might see them as criticism
❑ If all the participants are members of one organisation, they may have been influenced by its ideology and not recognise an outsider's interpretations
❑ Participants rely on their memory. They may not remember the meaning which they gave to a situation at the time
❑ If a long time has elapsed between the original *data collection* and the member check, participants may give a different interpretation to the phenomenon under study
❑ According to Ashworth (1993) member checks are not necessarily evidence of the trustworthiness of the research, because participants might not wish to disagree with the researcher

Nevertheless, member checks can enhance the trustworthiness of the findings, especially when a position of trust exists between the researcher and the participants.

MEMOING

Memoing is the construction of memos while carrying out qualitative research, in particular *grounded theory*. While going through the process of research, the researchers write memos. Strauss (1987) calls this 'memoing'. When observing and interviewing, the investigator writes *fieldnotes* from the beginning of the *data collection*. Certain occurrences or sentences seem of vital interest, and they are recorded either during or immediately after data collection. They remind the researcher of events, actions and interactions and trigger thinking processes.

There can be descriptions of the setting and written notes which are linked to the production of *theory*.

Memos are also reports on the analytic progress. They should be dated and detailed and are meant to help in the development and formulation of theory. In theoretical memos the researcher discusses tentative ideas and provisional *categories*, compares findings, and jots down thoughts on the research. Initially, memos might contain notes to remind the researcher, for example 'Don't forget...', or 'I intend to...'. Later they encompass micro-codes, and later still, major emergent categories, hunches, implications and concepts from the literature; memos become more varied and theoretical. Ideas for follow-up, related issues and thoughts about deviant cases become part of these memos. Strauss (1987) gives a number of different types of memos. Some of these are **preliminary**, and others are memos on **new categories** or **initial discovery** memos. (A complete list is given in Strauss, 1987.)

Strauss explains that memos are the written version of an internal dialogue going on during the research. Memos are provisional and can be changed as the research proceeds. Diagrams in the memos can help to remind the analyst and structure the study. Memoing continues throughout the whole of the research. It goes through stages and becomes more complex in the process. Memos and diagrams provide 'density' for the research and guide the researcher 'away from the data to abstract thinking, then in returning to the data to ground these abstractions in reality' (Strauss & Corbin, 1990: 199). Eventually, memos become integrated in the writing.

METAPHOR

A metaphor is a description imaginatively applied to a *phenomenon* but not actually true. Metaphors are rhetorical and representational devices that members of a *culture* use to share meaning and understanding (Coffey & Atkinson, 1996) and which contain figurative rather than literal language. The sentence 'I fought a battle against cancer' contains a metaphor.

While telling their *story*, participants use metaphors to enhance the understanding of their own lives. Burnard (1992) warns qualitative researchers not to take the use of metaphors too literally because it may lead to misinterpretation of the *data*. When listening to the conversations of *participants*, researchers must take care not to overlook them because of their familiarity.

Qualitative researchers themselves, too, use metaphors to enhance their writing and make it more lively. The *storyline* often improves and can be more easily grasped through the use of metaphors.

METHOD

Method consists of the procedures, strategies and techniques for the collection and analysis of data. It differs from *methodology*, a term that refers to the principles and *epistemology* on which researchers base their procedures and strategies.

METHOD SLURRING

This term, used by Baker, Wuest and Stern (Baker *et al.*, 1992), means a 'muddling' of different methods and procedures in a single piece of research.

Researchers cannot always differentiate between methods, and some expert researchers strongly argue against confusing them. Each approach in *qualitative research* has its own underlying principles, assumptions and procedures. The application differentiates methods and gives each approach its unique character (Morse, 1994). When using a particular method the researcher should make sure that language, philosophy and strategies 'fit' the chosen approach. Commonalities do exist, such as the focus on the experience and meanings of *participants*, the use of small samples and a strong *storyline*. Diverse pathways of qualitative research with different language use have been developed, although they cannot always be wholly separated from each other. Purposes and procedures differ. Delamont & Atkinson (1995) criticise the thinking inherent in the term 'method slurring', claiming that Baker, Wuest and Stern do not compare like with like. This can be seen below.

Grounded theory has as its aim the generation and development of theoretical ideas and focuses particularly on shared meanings in interaction. It is an approach to data collection and analysis, a style of research as Strauss (1987) calls it. *Data collection* and analysis interact and theoretical sampling is carried out until *saturation* occurs. Through *constant comparison* researchers uncover the social reality of participants. In the development of grounded theory, theorising is of particular importance.

Ethnography, on the other hand, is a study of *culture*. The first step for researchers is to become familiar with the setting they study and wish to research. The sample consists of key informants who possess special cultural knowledge.

Through finding patterns and themes, ethnographers uncover the rules and rituals of cultural members and write an ethnography to describe these.

Phenomenology is not a method as such but a philosophy. It explores the participants' 'lived experience' starting with their own reflections. Researchers select the sample on the basis of people's experiences or another important criterion. Through the *data*, *meanings* are found which demonstrate the characteristics of a phenomenon. Meaning units are translated into statements eventually forming the description of the phenomenon under study. Thus phenomenology gives authentic descriptions of experiences and phenomena. This resembles the research process inherent in the symbolic interactionist perspective and grounded theory described in other parts of this book. Approaches within the symbolic interactionist perspective focus on interaction while phenomenological researchers look at cognitive and affective phenomena (that is, thoughts and feelings).

Writers often describe an approach but do not develop in detail the procedures adopted, nor do they always describe the strategies used. Different methods originate in a variety of disciplines and tend to lack a single underlying set of theories (Atkinson, 1995). This does not necessarily mean the use of completely different procedures for each approach. Atkinson warns about 'prescriptive treatment' in the qualitative research process and 'tightly bounded typologies'. He does not believe in their exclusivity and claims that all qualitative methods do not belong to a single *paradigm*.

Modification of data collection and *data analysis* type is not only possible but can occasionally even be desirable and enhance creativity. This means breaking the rules and guidelines of specific approaches. Researchers should, of course, know about the assumptions and procedures of different qualitative methods. Then they can be flexible and modify their approach.

METHODOLATRY

Methodolatry (from *method* and idolatry) is a term used by Janesick (1994) to mean a preoccupation with method or overemphasis on method at the expense of content and storyline in *qualitative research*. Researchers are preoccupied with methodological concepts such as *validity* and *reliability* and neglect the *participants'* experience and interpretation. In qualitative research, method is often emphasised because researchers wish to make it respectable and acceptable in the world of research. Experimental research still seems to be regarded as the 'gold standard' in spite of its limitations in a sociocultural context.

METHODOLOGY

Methodology refers to the principles and philosophy on which researchers base their procedures and strategies, and to the assumptions that they hold about the nature of the research they carry out. It consists of the ideas underlying *data collection* and analysis. Methodology is more than *method*. The latter merely involves the procedures and techniques adopted by the researcher.

MODEL

A model is an abstract representation of reality. It involves a set of assumptions, constructs and relationships. Researchers can use it for analytical purposes as a 'simplification of complex reality' (Jary & Jary, 1991).

N

NARRATIVE

Narratives are stories which individuals tell about their condition, work or life. They are not new forms of *data collection* but have existed for centuries as autobiographies, diaries, oral histories or travellers' tales. In the past, narratives were not analysed systematically, nor did they always form part of a research approach. They have found a place in naturalistic inquiry because they are in tune with the world view of qualitative researchers. Narratives are especially useful for studying transformations and transitions in individuals' lives. Researchers analyse and search for *meaning* so that they transform the *story* from a journalistic report or literary text into research. Narratives are interpretations or modifications of reality, not merely a factual account of events. They are, according to Denzin (1989c), accounts of events and have a plot and a *storyline*. Researchers can focus on single cases – looking at the story of one individual – or multiple case studies through which they explore the lives of a group of people. Dickinson & Erben (1995: 254) call them 'patterns of stories' in the life experiences of people in their social *context*.

Narratives differ from unstructured interviews. The researcher lets the participants develop their tales and gives them long continuing stretches of time. The interviewer asks very few questions and encourages the participants to tell their own story, reconstruct it and relive their experiences. Through narratives and life histories, researchers can identify people's feelings, beliefs and actions, but only if they are thoughtful and sensitive listeners. Researchers learn how events from the past have influenced people.

Riessman (1993) distinguishes between three types of narrative.

❑ In a **habitual narrative**, routine events and actions are recalled
❑ **Hypothetical narratives** describe events which did not take place. An imaginary story would be an example of this
❑ A **topic-centred narrative** is a story of past events connected thematically by the storyteller.

Narratives are interpretations; while telling the story people give meaning to that which happened to them. These stories are given in simple natural language. Participants generally recall most vividly the events and actions that influenced them or made a strong impression. The person who has an experience tells a tale to the listener who was not there when it happened. The storytellers want to re-create past feelings and transmit them to other people. Ricoeur (1984, 1985) links narrative to temporality. Through narratives, past, present and often future are linked. This continuity is of great interest to qualitative researchers. Bruner (1987) explains that autobiographical accounts contain a selective record of events, 'reinterpretations' of life experiences which are 'constructed in people's heads'. Qualitative researchers wish to hear these stories in which people make sense of the past and present.

The narrative is a powerful medium through which researchers and readers can gain access to the world of participants and share their experiences. Examples of questions which encourage participants to report on their lives are, for instance: 'Tell me what happened', or 'Tell me about your feelings and thoughts at that time'. As in unstructured interviewing, open-ended questions are the most appropriate. (See also *life history*.)

NATIVE

A 'native' is an original member of the *culture* under study. The native need not be part of a strange or foreign culture but is often a member of a group in the researcher's own society. This term is not used as much now as in traditional social *anthropology*.

NATURALISM

In *qualitative research* this means the study of people in their natural environment, not in a controlled or laboratory situation. It is **inadvisable to use this term in qualitative research** as it often has a different interpretation in the social sciences (this is why the term 'naturalistic inquiry' is problematic). In natural science it means that people are part of nature and that the approach used to study their reality should be similar to that of the natural sciences.

NEGATIVE CASE

Negative cases are examples that do not fit into the working hypotheses of the researcher. **Negative case analysis** means searching for and analysing data that do not confirm the findings of the research so far and make the researchers revise their propositions. The search can only stop when the emerging ideas are not disconfirmed by a single case. Negative case analysis shows variation in the *data* and develops the study.

NOMOTHETIC

Using nomothetic *methods* means that researchers search for law-like generalities or rule-following behaviour which subsumes individual cases. (See also *idiographic*.)

O

OBJECTIVITY

To achieve objectivity is one of the aims of the researcher; it is seen as a sign of rigour. The notion of objectivity means that researchers do not let their own values or political stance impinge on the enquiry. Quantitative researchers in particular try to achieve objectivity by distancing themselves from respondents in order to avoid 'contamination' of the data. They assume that they can achieve the aim of 'scientific' inquiry by gaining objective knowledge, relatively free from *bias*. Qualitative researchers suggest that this view of science takes the world as consisting of measurable facts little affected by human beings. Objectivism, they claim, is impossible.

Research covers a continuum between relatively objective and subjective perspectives. Researchers carry out experiments, for instance, in which subjects or subject matter are randomly assigned to particular treatments or conditions, or they undertake surveys, using questionnaires or standardised interviews. The former are tightly controlled and often take place under laboratory conditions. They are generally seen as most objective because the researcher's values and background interfere least. In this type of research, biases are excluded as far as possible to obtain the 'truth'. The research report or study is generally written in the passive form or third person in this type of research. However, the idea that researchers can be completely objective is a myth, a fact which most researchers, regardless of their choice of methodology, now recognise.

The search for *objectivity* is problematic in all research. Objectivity in quantitative research emerges, so researchers claim, as a result of standardisation and distance from the respondents. Even this type of research cannot achieve complete objectivity and *value neutrality*: facts as seen by people are full of meaning; indeed researchers always bring their own values and ideas to the investigation. Choice of topic area, the type of *sampling* and the interpretation of *data* are affected by the researchers' perspectives and therefore contain elements of ***subjectivity***.

OBSERVATION

Observation is one of the strategies in *data collection*. Researchers as observers look at places and people in their natural settings. Qualitative researchers generally use 'participant observation', a term originally coined by Lindemann (1924).

Participant observation has its origins in *anthropology* and sociology. From the early days of *fieldwork*, anthropologists and sociologists became part of the *culture* they studied and examined the actions and interactions of people in their social context, 'in the field.' Famous studies in anthropology are those of Mead (1935) and Malinowski (1922) on other cultures; in sociology the participant observation of Strauss and his colleagues in psychiatric hospitals (Strauss *et al.*, 1964) and Spradley's work with tramps in the 1960s (Spradley, 1970) typify some of the early, well known studies.

Immersion in a setting is the first step in observation and can take a long time. **Prolonged engagement** in observation generates more in-depth knowledge of a culture or subculture, and researchers can avoid disturbances and potential biases caused by occasional visits. Observation is less disruptive and more unobtrusive than *interviews*. However, participant observation does not just involve observing the situation, but also listening to the people under study. Researchers can take any appropriate setting as a focus for their study. Participant observation varies on a continuum from open to closed settings. **Open settings** are public and highly visible, such as street scenes, hospital corridors and reception areas. In **closed settings**, access is difficult; doctors' surgeries, management meetings or clinics can be considered closed settings.

The participant observer enters the setting without intending to limit the observation to particular processes or people and adopts an unstructured approach. Occasionally certain foci crystallise early in the study, but usually observation progresses from the unstructured to the more focused until eventually specific actions and events become the main interest of the researcher. It is important to differentiate between significant and relatively unimportant *data* in the setting.

Gold (1958) identified four types of observer involvement in the field.

The four types of observer involvement in the field (Gold, 1958)
❑ The complete participant
❑ The participant as observer
❑ The observer as participant
❑ The complete observer

The complete participant

The complete participant is part of the setting and takes an insider role which often involves covert observation. Complete participation generates a number of problems. First, one would have to question seriously whether covert observation, particularly in teaching or care settings, without knowledge or permission of the people observed, is ethical. After all, this is not a public, open situation such as a street corner or rally, where nobody can be identified.

The participant as observer

Participants as observers have negotiated their way into the setting, and as observers they are part of the work group under study. For health workers or teachers this seems a good way of doing research as they are already involved in the work situation. Many nurses and midwives wish to examine a problem in their ward or in the hospital. Teachers often want to explore situations in their school. They then ask permission from the relevant gate-keepers and participants and explain their observer roles to them. The first advantage of this type of observation is the ease with which researcher–participant relationships can be forged or extended. Secondly, the observers can move around in the location as they wish, and thus observe in more detail and depth. For new researchers, observation is more difficult than interviewing because of the ethical issues involved. For instance, patients have to be protected from intrusion when interaction with health professionals is explored. To ask all patients in a particular ward to give permission to participate may be difficult but possible. *Ethics committees* are often reluctant, however, to allow young students to observe. It is easier for experienced researchers to gain *access*.

The observer as participant

The observer as participant is only marginally involved in the situation. For instance, health professionals might observe a ward in a hospital but do not directly work as part of the work force; they have, however, announced their interest and their public role and gone through the process of gaining *entry*. The advantage of this type of observation is the possibility for the professional to ask questions, to be accepted as a colleague and researcher but not to be called upon as a member of the work force. On the other hand, observers are prevented from playing a 'real' role in the setting, and this restraint from involvement is not easy, particularly in a busy work situation. Researchers must always ask permission from those in the setting.

The complete observer

Complete observers do not take part in the setting, and use a 'fly on the wall' approach. Observing behaviour in reception areas or in an accident and emergency department are examples of this. The complete observer situation is only possible when the researchers observe through a two-way mirror in a setting where they are not visible and have no impact on the situation. This strategy is commonly used in child guidance clinics in order to observe family interaction. Again, permission from participants should be asked.

Spradley (1980) claims that observers take three main steps: they use descriptive, focused and finally selective observation. Descriptive observation proceeds on the basis of general ideas that the observer has in mind. Everything that goes on in the situation becomes a source of data and is recorded, including colours, smells and appearances of people in the setting. Description involves all five senses. As time goes by, certain important areas or aspects of the setting become more obvious, and the researcher focuses on these because they contribute to the achievement of the aim of the research. Eventually the observation becomes highly selective.

LeCompte & Preissle (1993) list the different types of questions that can be asked in the observation.

Questions to ask in the observation

The 'who' questions
Who can be found in the setting, and how many people are present? What are their characteristics and roles?

The 'what' questions
What is happening in the setting, what are the actions and rules of behaviour? What are the variations in the behaviour observed?

The 'where' questions
Where do interactions take place? Where are people located in the physical space?

The 'when' questions
When do conversations and interactions take place? What is the timing of activities?

The 'why' questions
Why do people in the setting act the way they do? Why are there variations in behaviour?

Mini-tour observation leads to detailed descriptions of smaller settings, while grand-tour observations are more appropriate for larger settings. A study could take place in a hospital ward or the large urban hospitals in the country, in a classroom or in all schools in a county. After the initial stages, certain dimensions and features of observation become interesting to the researcher who then proceeds to observe these dimensions specifically. *Progressive focusing* is not just a feature of interviewing but also of observation. If researchers describe all activities and events, they will eventually distinguish what is important for the research from irrelevant details.

Focused observations are the outcome of specific questions. From broader observations researchers proceed to observing small units for investigation. The researchers look for similarities and differences among groups and individuals. For this type of observation a narrow focus and specificity are useful and necessary.

Marshall & Rossman (1995: 79) state that 'observation entails the systematic noting and recording of events, behaviours and artefacts (objects) in the social setting chosen for study'. The situation can then be analysed. Researchers observe social processes as they happen and develop. Although observers can examine events and ongoing actions, they cannot explore past events and thoughts of participants; this is only possible in interviews. Usually, though, interviewing is seen as part of participant observation. The study by Becker and his colleagues (1961) shows this clearly: they observed the participants, medical students, in their interaction with patients, colleagues and teachers and then asked questions about what they saw and heard. Hammersley & Atkinson (1995) propose that one might see all social research as participant observation insofar as the researcher actively participates in the situation.

Professionals sometimes shy away from formal participant observation because of problems of access, *ethics* and time. For instance, it is easier to obtain permission to interview colleagues than to observe them, because any observation would include observing clients. Observation might change the situation, as people act differently when they are observed although they often forget the presence of the observer in long-term observation.

When observations are successful, they can uncover interesting patterns and developments that have their basis in the real world of the participants' daily lives. The task of exploration and discovery is, after all, the aim of *qualitative research*. One of the advantages of observations is their immediacy. Researchers are able to reflect on events and actions as they occur in a particular *context* and do not have to rely on participants' accounts and reconstruction. Even the difference in 'what people say and what they do' (Deutscher, 1970) can become a source of data.

Covert observation

In covert observation researchers do not disclose the real reason for their presence in the setting. Many social researchers use these covert methods because they think their presence as researchers might produce *reactivity*, namely the observer effect, and that they can minimise it through covert observation. Some researchers feel that certain groups have something to hide, and they sometimes wish to examine exactly those types of behaviour and perspectives that are hidden from public view. Although this type of research might generate useful results, most qualitative researchers would see it as unacceptable due to ethical considerations, particularly in the health, social care and education fields.

Practical and ethical considerations

Researchers negotiate *access* with *gatekeepers* and participants. The *ethics* issues are similar to those in other types of qualitative research. All the people observed in a private setting should be asked for their permission for the study. The ethical issue is somewhat different in public settings such as a theatre, the street or another public place where observation can sometimes take place without permission for access. Ethical behaviour, however, is always expected from researchers.

When researchers study a social setting, they try to become part of the background so that they minimise the **observer effect**. Usually they take their place in a corner of the room to be as unobtrusive as possible. The corner is chosen to give maximum visual scope to the observer, but he or she should not be identified with any one group participating in the setting. Sanger (1996) also advises that researchers enter the location at the same time as the other people in the setting in order to draw minimal attention to themselves. Indeed, observation might be considered the least intrusive strategy because researchers often become part of the background.

ONTOLOGY

Ontology is a direction in philosophy concerned with the nature of being and existence. *Epistemology* and *methodology* are based on ontological questions covering, for example, the nature of social reality and assumptions about human existence. Ontological questions are a particular concern of *phenomenology* and participatory action research but are of importance in all research.

P

PARADIGM

A paradigm is a philosophical *model* or framework originating in a world view and belief system based on a particular *ontology* and *epistemology* and shared by a scientific community.

The *concept* has become popular through the writing of Thomas Kuhn (1970), the philosopher and historian of science, in his work *The Structure of Scientific Revolutions*. He believed that communities of scientists hold in common sets of assumptions and values, follow certain rules and fulfil certain expectations in their search for solutions to problems. Most scientists are involved in 'normal science' and work within the boundaries of this paradigm. There are, however, certain times in history when scientists become critical of existing beliefs and realise that problems cannot be solved within the paradigm of 'normal science'. Eventually a 'scientific revolution' and a 'paradigm shift' occurs when these scientists develop a fundamentally new framework based on different assumptions and new criteria for research. Eventually this paradigm too becomes 'normal science', and the cycle begins again.

Kuhn has influenced both natural and social science. Social scientists have taken his ideas and applied them to their research traditions. Some see *positivism* and *interpretivism* as different paradigms. Delamont & Atkinson (1995) criticise the 'paradigm wars'. They also deplore the 'paradigm mentality', particularly in education and nursing. These disciplines, they argue, recontextualise and simplify knowledge and theory originating in the social sciences. The theoretical, methodological and philosophical approaches of qualitative inquiry do not form a coherent whole. The rigid boundaries that educators and nurses establish and their insistence on paradigms have helped to create the myth of 'purity' and 'certainty' in qualitative research.

PARADIGM CASE

The paradigm case, a term used in phenomenological research (Benner, 1994), is an example of a specific pattern of *meaning*. It provides the knowledge to achieve understanding of the *participants'* behaviour and their interpretations of the world. Through these cases we are able to engage with the text. Researchers select the case that they think might best illustrate the *phenomenon* under study and explore and develop it. When one paradigm case has been described, others can then be examined and compared to the preceding case. In other words, paradigm cases allow for comparison of similarities and differences. The reason for the selection of a paradigm case should become clear to the reader of a research report.

PARTICIPANT

The participants in the research project are the people sampled, those whose perspectives researchers explore. Most qualitative researchers prefer the term 'participant', expressing the collaboration between the researcher and the researched (DePoy & Gitlin, 1993) and the equality of their relationship. This term, however, may be misleading as the researcher, too, is a participant.

Qualitative researchers favour the terms 'participant' or 'informant'. In surveys by structured interviews and written questionnaires, the most frequent term has been 'respondents'. Indeed, many qualitative researchers and research texts still use it (for instance Miles & Huberman (1994)), but it seems less frequent now in texts and reports about *qualitative research*.

Morse (1991b) claims that 'respondent' implies a passive response to the researcher's question which acts as a stimulus. Researchers' thinking influences the terms they use, and 'respondent' and 'subject' sound too mechanistic and passive in qualitative research. The terms researchers use make explicit their stance and their relationship to those being studied. Experimental and survey researchers refer to 'subjects'. This demonstrates the unequal position of researcher and researched.

Anthropologists refer to 'informants', those members of a *culture* or group who voluntarily 'inform' the researcher about their world and play an active part in the research. Morse usually chooses this term, though she acknowledges the suggestion by some journal editors that it might be seen to have links to the word 'informant' as used by the police. In the end, however, researchers must choose for themselves which term suits their research. In Morse's words: 'Subjects, respondents, informants, participants – choose your own term, but choose a term that fits' (Morse, 1991b: 406).

PEER DEBRIEFING

Peer debriefing is a process in which an outsider – another researcher, academic or professional – reviews the *data* and the analysis with the researcher who presents the problems and working hypotheses for discussion to this colleague. The process can start early at the design stage. It is useful because outsiders are not involved with the *data collection* or the *participants*, and they can examine the situation more dispassionately. Colleagues also provide the researchers with a listening ear and alleviate their isolation. Peer debriefing should not be carried out by a superior or a research supervisor because of the power relationships involved.

PHENOMENOGRAPHY

Phenomenography is a form of research that is related to *phenomenology*. The Swedish educationist, Ference Marton (1981, 1986) developed it initially in the 1970s with a group of researchers at the University of Gothenburg. Since then it has also been used in a number of other countries such as Australia. Phenomenography aims to describe phenomena and focuses on the under-standing and variations of experience within the social *context*. Phenomeno-graphers study conceptions of the world and the 'distinctively different ways' in which individuals understand, experience and interpret social phenomena.

PHENOMENOLOGY

Phenomenology is a philosophical approach to the study of 'phenomena' (appearances) and human experience. It is a philosophy and an attitude to human existence and not a research method, but it has been used as a *method* to explore the **lived experience** of people. Although phenomenology is still one of the most important schools of philosophy in the twentieth century, it does not seem to have developed as a dominant philosophy in recent years (Cohen, 1987). It has had an impact on philosophical thinking and served as a basis for *qualitative research*, particularly in the areas of health and illness (Oiler Boyd, 1993; Benner, 1994; Streubert & Carpenter, 1995); in psychology (Vallé & King, 1978, Giorgi, 1985) and, to a lesser extent, in educational inquiry (van Manen, 1990). To understand the place of phenomenology in qualitative research, it is important to examine its development.

The development of phenomenology

Spiegelberg's (1960) work is still seen as the definitive document on the history of the phenomenological movement. He describes the history of phenomenology as consisting of three stages: the preparatory phase, the German phase and the French phase.

Franz Brentano (1838–1917) presents the early stage of the movement, the 'preparatory phase' providing the groundwork for later phenomenology. He was the first to stress the 'intentional nature of consciousness' and developed the concept of **intentionality** which Moustakas (1994: 28) describes as referring to consciousness, 'to the internal experience of being conscious of something' (intentionality here has specialised meaning, not to be confused with the common-sense concept). Brentano saw intentionality as an important aspect in the study of mental phenomena and claimed that consciousness is always directed at an object; for instance, awareness or perception are always awareness and perception of something. Brentano set the goals of phenomenology: that philosophy answer questions about the concerns of humanity, and to develop a scientific, descriptive psychology.

The second and most important stage of phenomenology is the German phase initiated by the German philosopher Edmund Husserl (1859–1938) who was Brentano's student. Husserl, too, believed in phenomenology as a rigorous science and in the notion of intentionality.

Husserl developed the concepts of intuition, essence, phenomenological reduction and intersubjectivity. '**Intuiting**' or intuition (*Anschauung*) is an element of Husserl's philosophy. He believed in the phenomenologist's intuitive understanding of human experience. Human beings describe the phenomena they observe and interpret them. **Intuition** demands that the observer becomes immersed in the object of his or her perception and relates it to other phenomena. Intuiting can also go on in the memory or the imagination.

Stripping away the everyday, going to the very foundations of things, human beings are able to recognise essences, the 'real', 'intended' meanings of phenomena under investigation. Husserl wanted to get through to the **essence** or **eidos** of a phenomenon he believed open to intuition. Accurate description of phenomena is therefore important. He was not a relativist but believed in absolute and universal truths about human existence.

Husserl developed the concept of **phenomenological reduction**. In this, things and phenomena are viewed without prior judgement or assumptions; they are seen and described as they appear through *observation* and experience. This means going to 'the things themselves'. The mathematical term **bracketing** is used for this suspension of preconceptions. To be able to bracket, individuals have first to make explicit their preconceptions and suppositions so that these are clear and understandable even by themselves. Complete reduction, however, is never possible (Merleau-Ponty, 1962).

The terms *intersubjectivity* and life-world were mainly developed by Husserl's students and co-workers. Husserl's interest is in the structure of the **life-world** (Lebenswelt), the **lived experience** of people whose environment is not separate or independent from them. **Intersubjectivity** means that human beings live in a shared world. Every person is imbued with the sense of 'the Other' and has access to the experience of others through his or her own personal experience.

The philosopher Martin Heidegger (1889–1976) was concerned with Being and Time (this was also the title of his major work in 1927). He was interested in the nature of the self as 'Being-in-the world', which means that people's existence is always connected with the world in which they live. The two cannot exist without each other, and a continuous dialogue goes on between the person and his or her world; the person and the world 'co-constitute' each other. Heidegger's concept of *Dasein* (Being there) focuses on the nature of being, on the idea of personhood and on temporality.

Heidegger influenced the third phase in phenomenology, the French phase including Gabriel Marcel (1889), Jean Paul Sartre (1905–1980) and Maurice Merleau-Ponty (1908–1961). Marcel, a writer, saw phenomenology as an important basis for the analysis of being and existence, and he provided the later ideas for the philosopher Merleau-Ponty. The writer, Sartre, was a phenomenological existentialist. He too developed the concept of intentionality. His main ideas focus on the tragedy of human existence (the title of one of his books, first published in 1943, is: *Being and Nothingness* (Sartre, 1965)) and the concept of freedom to which human beings are 'condemned'. Merleau-Ponty (1962) tried to show the importance of individual experience and examined 'perception' as a significant part of a science of human beings. Like other phenomenologists, he was critical about the positivist concept of science that neglects subjective experience and stresses *objectivity*. Existential phenomenologists such as Sartre and Merleau-Ponty do not believe that existence can be bracketed.

Phenomenological analysis

As stated, phenomenology is not a research method in itself, hence researchers who use this approach are reluctant to describe specific techniques. They fear that the strategies might be seen as rules and become inflexible (Hycner, 1985). They focus instead on attitude and the response to the phenomenon under study. The aim is phenomenological description. This is an analytic description of the phenomena not affected by prior assumptions. The description – which Colaizzi (1978) calls 'perceptual description' – directly presents the rich experience of the participants. Phenomenological research focuses on what it means to be human. Phenomenological description can never encompass the whole of the phenomenon but shows only particular aspects, including hidden meanings, and these are always the meanings of the people under study. The phenomenologist has to go beneath the surface and beyond appearances. The data are obtained through *interviews* or the *narratives* of the participants. The language, facial expressions and gestures of the people interviewed are noted during the research.

Some of the better known phenomenological researchers and teachers of research methods are Giorgi *et al.* (1971), Colaizzi (1978) and van Manen (1984, 1990).

Colaizzi's seven steps of phenomenological analysis are an example of strategies used in phenomenology on a practical level.

(1)   After interviewing participants and transcribing the data, researchers repeatedly read the participants' descriptions and listen to the tapes to become familiar with their words. Through these processes they gain the feeling inherent in participants' meanings and a 'sense of the whole'. Giorgi (1975) calls this the 'Gestalt', the unified form.

(2)   Researchers then return to the participants' descriptions and focus on those aspects that are seen as most important for the phenomenon under study. Every sentence and paragraph is scrutinised for significant statements. These statements are isolated and expressed in general formulations. For instance: 'I always listened to the nurse; she was important to me; after all, she knew about my condition', becomes: 'Trust in professional opinion and advice'. Colaizzi called this step of isolating important sayings '**extracting significant statements**'.

(3)   Colaizzi calls this stage **formulating meanings**. The researcher takes each significant statement and makes sense of it in the participants' own terms. Hidden meanings are uncovered.

(4)   The processes are repeated for each interview, and the meanings are organised into **clusters of themes**. Common patterns tend to become obvious when this step is taken. Researchers take the clusters of *themes* back to the data so that they can confirm and validate the emerging patterns. The process of examining the data in the light of emerging themes has to be repeated until everything is accounted for.

(5)   Colaizzi calls this step **exhaustive description**. It is a detailed, analytic description of the participants' feelings and ideas contained in the themes.

(6)   The researcher then formulates an exhaustive description of the area under study and identifies its **fundamental structure**.

(7)   The last step consists of a ***member check*** (sometimes called respondent validation) in which the findings are taken back to the participants. These are asked to add what the researcher omitted to capture in the data so that it can be included in the final version of the study. Hycner (1985) advises researchers to summarise each interview, including the themes that were found, and to show them to the participant so that ideas can be modified or new ideas added.

Giorgi and van Kaam, two members of the Duquesne School of Phenomenology (from Duquesne University) also developed their own styles of analysis which are not the same as but similar to Colaizzi's (see Crotty, 1996: 22–3). A common characteristic is the concern with developing themes from the data which form the basis of 'exhaustive description' or the description of the 'whole' phenomenon.

Researchers should read with an open mind and suspend prior assumptions by making them explicit and being aware of them. They follow the ideas of the participants rather than imposing their own. Hycner (1985) adds that researchers' peers can verify the meanings implicit in the words of the participants. Colleagues are asked to examine the findings (*peer debriefing*). When there is agreement about the meaning, it can be assumed that the original researcher has bracketed his or her assumptions, and therefore the research is seen as more rigorous. Hycner advocates that themes which deviate from the general pattern should also be discussed in the study.

Sampling in phenomenological research progresses in a similar way to other qualitative research. The sample is taken from those with experience of the condition or knowledge of the phenomenon. Because of the depth of the research interviews and their analysis, the sample is generally very small. There is no control group.

There is great diversity in the phenomenological movement. Phenomenology in sociology was developed initially by Alfred Schütz (1899–1959) who wrote *The Phenomenology of the Social World* in 1932 (published here in 1967). Applying Husserl's ideas to social phenomena, he was concerned with typifications and intersubjectivity: social *actors* construct their world together and have 'taken for granted assumptions' about it because of a reciprocity of perspectives. They organise their world by creating typical traits of people or events. Typification relies on the classification system of researchers: for instance, Stockwell (1984) showed that nurses might group patients into popular and unpopular patients.

This is an example of typification. Social interaction proceeds on the basis of these typifications which have their roots in the 'stock of knowledge at hand'. Schütz had a particular influence on *ethnomethodology*.

Phenomenological researchers try to comprehend the essences of phenomena. They stress that the participant is a person and a unique human being who nevertheless shares this humanity with others and is linked to the world. (Moustakas (1994: 180) has a simple outline as a model for phenomenological research.)

PILE SORTING

This is a technique in which ethnographers present a list of items on cards to the *participants* and ask them for similarities, differences or other relationships between them (Hudelson, 1994). The technique is similar to *card sorting*. Researchers ask participants to sort cards into piles according to criteria that have *meaning* for them. Then participants explain the grouping of cards. As researchers do not wish to impose ideas on the participants, they generally use the technique of *free listing* prior to pile sorting.

PILOT STUDY

A pilot study is a small-scale trial run of the research with a very small number of participants chosen by the same criteria as those in the research. It is exploratory. Problems can be discovered and avoided when the research starts. While pilots are essential in quantitative research, in qualitative approaches pilot studies are not necessary because the research has the flexibility for the researcher to 'learn on the job' (Robson, 1993). The small number of cases, too, makes pilot studies difficult because there may not be enough informants who fulfil the criteria demanded for the sampling in the pilot study. Piloting can be carried out if the researcher lacks confidence or is a novice, particularly when using the interview technique.

PORTRAIT WRITING

Where the researcher paints a portrait in words (Bogdan & Biklen, 1992) the term 'portrait writing' is used. This occurs often in qualitative research when writers wish to tell a lively story. Bogdan and Biklen attribute this term to Denny (1978).

POSITIVISM

Positivism is an approach to science based on the natural science model in which a belief in universal laws and law-like generalities can be found. One of the rules in this type of research is the quest for *objectivity* and neutrality so that distance can be preserved and personal biases avoided. Investigators searched for patterns and regularities and believed that universal laws and rules or law-like generalities exist. They thought that *generalisability* – possible application to other situations and cases – would be possible if random sampling is used.

Positivists followed the natural science approach in which theories and hypotheses are tested and verified or falsified. They insisted on neutrality and objectivity. Science was seen as neutral and value-free; that is, scientists do not adopt a moral or political stance. The methods of natural – in particular physical – science stem from the eighteenth and nineteenth centuries. Comte (1798–1857), the French philosopher, suggested that the newly emerging social sciences must proceed in the same way as natural science by adopting the natural science method of observation and experimentation as opposed to speculation or theological explanations of phenomena. Much social research is based on the positivist and early natural science paradigm that has influenced social science throughout the nineteenth and the first half of the twentieth centuries. Behaviour could be predicted, so researchers believed, on the basis of universal law-like generalities. Even today many researchers think that at the heart of all research lie numerical measurement, statistical analysis and the search for cause and effect. They feel that detachment and objectivity are possible, and that numerical measurement results in objective knowledge. In this approach, the researchers control the theoretical framework, the sampling frames and the structure of the research. Qualitative researchers who accept an interpretive model (see *interpretivism*) criticise this view of science. The danger of the positivist approach is that researchers treat perceptions of the social world as objective and absolute and neglect everyday subjective interpretations and the context of the research.

Post-positivism is a more recent direction in science in which positivist ideas have been modified and reformulated in a limited way to the criticism made of positivism although post-positivists still hold essentially similar beliefs. The difference lies in post-positivists' assumptions that there cannot be complete objectivity or truth, but that findings are probably true if all procedures to establish *validity* have been followed. It is therefore important that researchers view the findings critically and not as absolute and once-and-for-all. Post-positivists also accept that research cannot be completely value-free.

Popper (1959) – who did not see himself as a positivist – claimed that **falsifiability** of a *theory* is the main criterion of science. The researcher for-mulates a *hypothesis* – an expected outcome – and tests it. Consecutive findings help to confirm or reject the hypothesis, but any statement must always be falsifiable. If it is disproved, the whole process starts anew. Particular cases have to 'fit' the hypothesis. If 'fit' exists and the hypothesis is not falsified, the study is finished until the moment a deviant case occurs. Knowledge is always pro-visional. The main aim of this type of research is to test theory. This means that the approach develops from theory, and the concepts are established before the research begins. The *model* of science adopted is hypothetico-deductive.

In the 1960s the traditional view of science was attacked and criticised by both social and natural scientists, for its aims and methods, its emphasis on social reality as being 'out there' separate from the individual. Natural scientists – for instance biologists and physicists – do not agree exactly on what science is and adopt a variety of different scientific methods. They, too, criticise the mechanistic view of the world. Traditionalists believed that scientific know-ledge can be proven and is discovered by rigorous methods of observation and experiment and derived through the senses, a simplistic view of science (Chalmers, 1982). Scientific knowledge is difficult to prove and is not merely derived from the senses. The search for *objectivity* may be futile for scientists; they strive for it, but their own biases, experiences and opinions intrude.

Many social scientists claim that reality is socially constructed and defined (see *social constructionism*). *Meaning* is produced by human beings who interpret the natural and the social world. They resurrected the *interpretive* perspective which initially stemmed from the writings of Mead and others in the early century. This relates to some of the ideas of the sociologist Weber (1864–1920) and his ideas of *Verstehen*.

POSTMODERNISM

Postmodernism (or postmodernity) is a cultural phenomenon and stresses the plurality and diversity of values and beliefs. The main features of post-modernism are *relativism* and extreme *subjectivity*. Postmodernists do not believe in an absolute 'truth' and the scientific goal of predicting and controlling.

Postmodern researchers – which include, for instance, some phenomenologists and some feminists – reject the idea of causality and have doubts about the *generalisability* of knowledge. Indeed the scientific model of knowledge and ideas about truth are replaced by a model stressing myths and symbols. They transgress the boundaries between the arts and the sciences and often emphasise 'style, not content'. In research that adopts postmodern perspectives, the researchers' ideas are seen as no more valid than the ideas of others. The research report is often presented in an unconventional form such as a film, a poem or a play in line with the belief that perceptions of the world are achieved through representations and images rather than reality.

PREMATURE CLOSURE

Premature closure (Lincoln & Guba, 1985) means making inferences that are not based on all the evidence contained in the *data* or are arrived at too early in the research process. Researchers might interpret the data too quickly without examining them thoroughly or use *concepts* and *categories* that they have previously discovered or studied and try to fit these to the data at hand. The danger exists that once researchers have generated some theoretical ideas, they sit back and decide that they have arrived at full explanations for the phenomenon under study. Sometimes there has been no complete investigation or *data analysis*, sometimes researchers close their minds to new ideas; they fail to go from a simple to a more abstract level of analysis. The researcher must return to the data continually to check that all the ideas which they contain are represented in the emergent theory. Premature closure can lead to 'immature' theory, as Morse & Field (1996) believe.

PROGRESSIVE FOCUSING – or FUNNELLING

The process of interviewing or *observation* starts with a broad basis and becomes progressively more specific during the interview or observation process. Through progressive focusing researchers home in on particular selected topics and questions which are more important for the research than others.

PROPOSAL

A proposal (the term 'protocol' is often used in medical and biological research) is a detailed description of a proposed piece of research. This **plan of action** has to convince the reviewers that the researcher knows enough to conduct the research and can describe what he or she wishes to understand or learn. The proposal aims to clarify the research to funding agencies, official *gatekeepers* such as managers, *ethics committees*, and, for student work, to supervisors and tutors. Researchers explain what they will research, why they adopt a particular focus, and how they will proceed. (See Locke *et al.*, 1993.)

Proposals for most types of research follow similar guidelines, but qualitative researchers adopt more flexible procedures as the design develops during the course of the research. Although there should be a clear aim, a detailed statement of objectives is not necessary because they will emerge during the conduct of the research. A qualitative project does not need a *hypothesis*, though working hypotheses arise during the research. The number of individuals in the sample cannot be decided from the start in all types of qualitative research – for instance in *grounded theory* where theoretical sampling is used. A full description of the *methodology* is important.

Elements of a proposal for a qualitative research project

The proposal for a qualitative research project, similar to that for quantitative work, consists of the following main elements:

Title
Abstract
Introduction
    Problem statement and rationale (justification for the study)
    Context and setting
    The aim of the research
    The possible benefit for the service or business for which the research is
        intended (there may, of course, be an intellectual outcome only)
Initial literature review
    (A discussion of other researchers' work which demonstrates the need for
        the proposed study)
Methodology
    Theoretical basis and justification of the methodology
    Sample selection and sampling procedures
    Data collection and strategies
    Data analysis
Ethical and *entry* issues

(contd)

Timeline (time scale, timetable) of the proposed research
Finance and resources (for funded research: justification of the budget)
Dissemination
(For funded research: the curriculum vitae (CV) of each individual involved in the research)

The proposal should be clearly structured and the sections headed. Most researchers follow more or less the suggested guidelines, although reviewers (agencies, supervisors or *ethics committees*) might have their own format for the proposal. The main element of the proposal is coherence; its parts should be linked so that it makes sense to the readers.

Title

The *title* should reflect the aim of the research. In funded research a title is often provided by agencies, but students can usually choose their own. It should be concise (not more than about 16 words) but still provide an idea of the essence of the research.

Abstract

The *abstract* (or summary) of the research proposal is a very brief summary of the focus, aim and methods of the research. The abstract is written last although it precedes the other elements of the proposal. The proposal abstract should not take more than 100 words (sometimes no more than half this is necessary although an abstract for the final report takes between 150 and 250). The abstract is a short plan of the proposal.

Introduction

This section sets the scene for the research. In the introduction researchers demonstrate the quality and feasibility of the study and the reasons for it. Readers can only understand the proposal in the *context* in which the research is placed.

The introduction consists of

(1)   the problem statement and rationale
(2)   a statement of the aim of the research

The problem statement and rationale

Researchers briefly describe the research focus. Students and researchers who do not conduct commissioned research also show how they became aware of the problem, and explain why they want to find out about it. It is important that the research problem is not trivial but has significance and benefits for the particular industry or service for which it is conducted (or that it is important for its own sake).

Those researchers who are not constrained by their commissioning or funding bodies can address a new problem which occurred in the setting or adopt a new approach to a familiar problem. The rationale gives the reasons for the research which have often emerged through observation of a problem in a particular situation or were stimulated by reading about an event, a crisis or question in the clinical or community setting. At this stage researchers can mention some of the claims and suggestions that other writers make about the topic or area of study. The investigation of the problem should fill a gap in professional knowledge, however small that gap may be. The rationale is the justification for the selection of the problem and topic.

The aim

The aim of the study, a statement of the researcher's intentions, is made explicit. A broad statement of the aim is sufficient although some researchers give a general aim and a series of more specific objectives or steps to reach this aim. In qualitative research specific objectives might rigidify the study. If objectives must be given, the researcher should be prepared to change them in the course of the research. The aim of a qualitative study is non-directional and provides a general sense of the main idea using terms such as 'explore', 'develop', 'describe'. The statement of the study's aim does not contain more than a maximum of 25 words so it does not become convoluted and too complex.

The literature

The literature demonstrates the amount and level of knowledge that exists in the area of research. It is important to mention not only seminal research on the subject but also the most recent. Qualitative research is particularly appropriate when little is known about the area of research, because the researcher does not start with preconceived ideas.

In a qualitative literature overview the discussion of the literature tends to be less detailed than in other types of research. As the data have primacy, qualitative researchers tend to avoid taking too much direction from the literature, and in consequence they only discuss a few major research studies and demonstrate where the proposed project fills a gap in knowledge. The rest of the literature will become part of the data and will be integrated in the final project.

The methodology
The methodology section consists of

(1)   A rationale for its use
(2)   Sampling procedures
(3)   Data collection
(4)   Data analysis
(5)   Validity and reliability (or trustworthiness and authenticity if these terms are chosen)
(6)   The limitations of the study
(7)   The dissemination of the study

Rationale for the methodology
Methodology is concerned with the ideas and principles on which procedures are based. Researchers must identify, describe and justify the methodology they adopt and the strategies and procedures involved. It is, of course, important that the methods fit the research question. Some of the details of a qualitative research project cannot be pre-specified, because they arise during the research process.

Sampling procedures
Researchers describe the sampling strategies and explain the criteria for the selection of the sample. If these include theoretical sampling, for instance, this should also be explained. The sample size (or initial sample size) must be given and the target population from which the sample is chosen identified. Inclusion and exclusion criteria for the sample are outlined at this stage. The reader of the proposal should understand how the researcher recruited the participants and obtained access to them.

Data collection
Researchers describe how the data collection will proceed, for instance through in-depth interviews, participant observation, etc.

Data analysis
The data analysis is described in a few paragraphs. Researchers should also demonstrate that ethical issues have been considered.

Validity and reliability
Researchers describe how they make sure that the findings of the research are trustworthy and authentic.

Limitations of the study
Researchers outline the constraints and *limitations* of the project, and state how they would overcome them. Limitations are weaknesses in the research. By stating these and solutions to them, researchers show their careful preparation for the study. For example, one of the limitations of qualitative research is the lack of generalisibility; this must be acknowledged. It can be explained, however, how the lack of generalisability need not be a problem by describing attempts to achieve typicality or specificity.

Dissemination
Researchers identify the readership for whom they write and explain the usefulness of the study for the particular group they address. They can state how they will disseminate the results of the study, be it through journals, books or other media such as conferences and video and audio tapes.

Timetable
Reviewers wish to see a **timeline** for the research to examine its feasibility. Therefore qualitative researchers submit a projected work schedule for the research even though they cannot always predict exactly how long each step is going to take. All the steps are recorded on the timeline. This can be drawn as a diagram. **The analysis of data in qualitative research takes a long time**. It must become clear from the time scale that data collection and analysis proceed at the same time and interact, and that there is an ongoing process of searching the literature.

Resources
Researchers specify the use of resources and other costs to demonstrate that the research can be adequately funded. Resourcing and costs are important in proposals for grant-giving bodies and must be detailed. These include clerical costs, paper, and mailing as well as the researcher's time. Researchers rarely cost a computer because they usually work in institutions such as universities or research agencies where computers are readily available. Some funding agencies will not pay for a computer or the researcher's time.

It is a good idea to look at one's own proposal in the light of an evaluation checklist.

PROPOSITION

A proposition is a conclusion about the links between concepts. A proposition in qualitative research can be a *working hypothesis*, a provisional hypothesis which could be tested out in the process of the research.

PSEUDONYM

Pseudonyms are the names given to the informants of the study by the researcher or by themselves. They are fictitious names and should never be similar to the real names of the participants to safeguard anonymity. In a qualitative study researchers give a name to each *participant* to make the study more lively and interesting; a number might disturb the *storyline*. Sometimes it is useful to start with the letter in the alphabet that has the same number as the participant, for instance, participant 1 might be called Anna or Mrs Anders, participant 5 is named Edward or Mr Erben. This way researchers can tell immediately at which stage of the process they interviewed the person mentioned. On very rare occasions, when all participants wish to be identified by their own names, the researcher might decide not to use pseudonyms; however, this is very unusual.

Morse & Field (1996) advise against the use of names or even pseudonyms for fear that the participants' anonymity be threatened. Of course, researchers must take care that informants cannot be identified. None the less, researchers should demonstrate to the reader that they do not just use quotes from a few individual participants but have established general patterns and themes from all informant interviews. This they can do best by the use of pseudonyms while making sure of anonymity.

Q

QUALIDATA

QUALIDATA is the name of the Archival Resource Centre in the Department of Sociology in Essex set up by Professor Paul Thompson, now its director, and other members of the department. It was funded by the *ESRC*, the Economic and Social Research Council (for Britain), initially for five years from 1994. A number of subject disciplines are represented such as health studies, business studies, sociology, social policy, anthropology, education, history, political science, geography and social psychology (Corti *et al*., 1996).

QUALITATIVE RESEARCH

Qualitative research is an inclusive and wide-ranging term. Under its umbrella a number of methodologies, philosophies, methods and procedures can be found. These include: various types of *ethnography*, *grounded theory*, *phenomenology*, qualitative *case-study* methods, many types of textual analysis (for instance *conversation analysis* and *discourse analysis*), as well as some forms of action research and feminist standpoint research. Indeed these different approaches are not always wholly separate but may overlap. All these methods of inquiry, however, are part of the interpretive approach. (See *interpretivism*.)

QUESTIONING

Questioning in qualitative research involves asking questions during *interviews* or occasionally while observing a setting and situation. Researchers use different types of questions depending on the research topic and purpose.

Grand-tour questions involve broad overviews about larger topic areas. They elicit descriptions and stories about issues, routines and stages of participants' lives without restrictions and in a general form. Researchers often start with these and then go on to more specific and narrower areas. **Mini-tour questions** differ from grand-tour questions in their specific and narrow focus.

They specify a particular happening, a situation, an incident, a time or a rule, but they are also follow-ups and clarification (Spradley, 1979).

Interview questions are different from *research questions*. The former are specific and aim to produce the data about events and behaviour while research questions provide an overview of what the researcher wishes to learn or understand.

QUOTES

Quotes are verbatim statements (sentences or phrases) from interview participants. In a qualitative report they are integrated in the discussion of the findings and become part of the *storyline*. Interviewers extract the *meaning* of the quotes and interpret it for the reader who had no direct *access* to the participants and has to rely on the researcher who has first-hand and intimate knowledge of the data.

Researchers use quotes for the following reasons:

❑ to confirm and support the findings of the research and claims that are made
❑ to help the reader understand where categories or themes originate and how the researcher came to interpret the *data*
❑ to illustrate the experiences of the participants and their perceptions and feelings
❑ to enliven the report in order to advance the storyline and capture the interest of the reader

The function of quotes is not only to indicate an individual's specific experiences but also to demonstrate and give examples of patterns that have emerged in the research. Researchers do not choose words willy-nilly but carefully select those sections of participant talk which best represent the general ideas expressed in the report as well as the informant's specific interpretation. Researchers select the quotes that represent the informants' ideas on a specific topic area. The quotes are instances of a point made in the research report and illustrate the arguments (Sandelowski, 1994). The writers choose representative sections from the informants' words. Quotes never stand on their own but are linked to the *context* in which they occur and the claim which the researchers wish to make. This way, they provide evidence for their assertions. Although quotes from participants have their origin in the interviews, when used in the text they have already been interpreted by their very selection and do not stay 'raw' data. Great care should be taken not to take quotes out of context and mislead the reader about their meaning.

The number and length of quotes used in the report depend on the target and type of the research. The number of quotes illustrating an assertion or a statement of the researcher may be small in a report for a professional or grant-giving body. Journal editors, too, have their own ideas of the length, type and place of quotes. In a thesis or dissertation more are generally interwoven, but writers must take care not to spoil the storyline with strings of quotes on each page.

The participants' words should be used verbatim, though irrelevant comments or sentences can be removed. This is indicated by three dots, ... When laughter, crying or long silences occur, this is identified in the quote and surrounded by square brackets: [laughter] or [long pause]. Finally, the researcher must be careful that the informants cannot be identified from the quotes as the number of participants in *qualitative research* is often small.

When the quotes are typed, longer sentences or paragraphs are generally indented on both sides and more closely spaced than the rest of the text (if the text spacing is 2, the quote spacing might be 1½). No quotation marks are needed in this case. The longer quotes should be accompanied by an indication of the participant's *pseudonym* or *identifier* in words or numbers, for example (Nurse Atkinson), (Andrea), (Participant A) or (P 1).

Morse & Field (1996) advise against the use of names or pseudonyms for fear that the participants' anonymity may be threatened. Of course, researchers must take care that informants cannot be identified. None the less, researchers should demonstrate to the reader that they do not just use quotes from a few individual participants but have established general patterns and *themes* from all informant *interviews*. This they can do best by the use of *pseudonyms* while making sure of anonymity.

R

REACTIVITY

Reactivity is the reaction of the people studied to the research and the presence of the researcher. Reactivity is reflected in the observer effect and the interviewer effect.

The **observer effect** is an influence on the research which researchers produce through their expectations, predisposition and sometimes through their mere presence in the situation under study. *Participants* react to the presence of outsiders, and the setting itself may change through the observer effect. The **interviewer effect** is similar to the observer effect. Participants react to the researcher. As they might wish to please or to be seen in positive way, they might unconsciously or consciously tell lies or modify their answers to questions.

Hammersley & Atkinson (1995) advise researchers to adopt a **monitoring process** to recognise and minimise reactivity. They also claim, however, that reactivity can become a resource for researchers because the reaction of participants informs about their thoughts and feelings. Reactivity can be decreased through prolonged *observation* and full immersion in the situation so that participants get used to the presence of the researcher; nevertheless researchers should realise that the setting itself may change forever through their presence because participants become aware of their own practices.

Reflexivity about a researcher's presence and relationships in the setting has to be built into the research; for instance, official and unofficial accounts produce different dimensions and affect the emerging concepts and theories.

REALISM

Realism is the belief that a reality exists independent of the perceptions of human beings, and an assumption of objective reality. Some realists claim that both the physical and social worlds have a reality apart from human perceptions; others assume that only the physical, material world exists independently but not the social. Hammersley (1990: 61) rejects the claim of 'naive realism': the belief in a reality independent of human beings of which they have direct and certain knowledge. He advocates instead a more subtle realist approach. (See also *idealism*.)

RECORDING DATA

Researchers often record the *data* in a number of ways. They use **audio tapes** to record the words of the *participant*. Data can also be recorded by **video recorder**. The video tapes are a rolling picture of the research and are able to capture in detail the events and actions in the setting. Movement, stance and facial expressions as well as rule following and rituals can be recorded. As it is important to grasp the *context* in *qualitative research*, video recording is a good way in which the context boundedness is recorded, but audio recording is more common. Tapes are the most accurate records of data.

A technical manual for fieldworkers exists which describes the details of audio and video recording (Ives, 1995). Most qualitative researchers use common sense, try out their machines before starting recording and make sure that they have extra batteries if they are not connected to the mains. They should ensure that the tape is audible and visible by placing it in a convenient position, but not so near that the participants are intimidated. However, most people tend to forget the microphone and the camcorder during the research. Permission for taping is sought from each participant before an audio tape or video recorder can be installed.

Films, **photographs** or even drawings can be records for qualitative researchers in a similar way to videos. Photographs are particularly useful when researchers carry out historical qualitative research. (See *data sources*.)

REFLEXIVE JOURNAL

A reflexive journal or diary is the ongoing account of the researcher's pathways and decisions during the research and contains insights and reflections. Lincoln & Guba (1985) advise that this record should be used as part of the *audit trail*.

REFLEXIVITY

Researchers are reflexive when they refer back and critically examine their own assumptions and actions through being 'self-conscious' and self-aware about their research process. This **monitoring process** includes reflection about their reaction to the people and events in the setting. In practical terms this means that they might reflect on their relationship with the *participants*. They also examine the way they feel while carrying out the research and the effects of their *observations* on the people under study. They give reasons for their decisions to the readers of their report. Reflexivity is essential for qualitative research because the researcher is the main research tool; he or she 'uses the self as an instrument'.

W.J. Potter (1996) lists three strategies of reflexivity. In the first, the researcher gives details of the research process and the *context* of the research (see also *audit trail*). The second technique involves the author of the report in a reflection on the *methods* while taking a self-critical stance towards the interpretation of the data. The third consists of the disclosure of assumptions and *biases*.

It is important to realise that researchers are part of the reality they investigate, and they should reflect about their own location in *culture*, time and place. They will be conscious of their actions and interactions as well as about the roles they have in the field. Qualitative inquiry is affected by the social location of the researchers, their personalities and their values. Researchers are aware of, and reflect on, their own preconceptions and assumptions while attempting to understand the effect they have on the data. The process of reflection also uncovers contradictions and paradoxes.

RELATIVISM

Relativism is a theoretical approach which claims that objective knowledge does not exist, but that knowledge depends on the social environment and the perceptions of people. It is seen as relative and socially constructed. Different aspects and views of reality can only be judged relative to each other and not in relation to an objective truth. Reality depends on the person who created it or the group and *culture* sharing it. Many researchers with an interpretivist or hermeneutic approach take a relativist stance, but social scientists often criticise extreme relativism (Hammersley, 1990). Silverman (1993) points out that it ultimately prevents individuals from adopting any stance at all.

RELIABILITY

Reliability is the extent to which a technique or procedure will generate the same results regardless of how, when and where the research is carried out or the extent to which the instrument is consistent. The term cannot be used in an absolute sense. This consistency is difficult to achieve in qualitative research because the researcher is the main research instrument. (See also *replicability* and *validity*.)

REPLICABILITY

Replicability exists when a researcher adopts the same procedures with a similar sample and setting used by another researcher and obtains similar findings, that is when the research is repeatable. One of the tenets of science is that the results of the research are replicable. Qualitative research cannot be replicated in the same way as quantitative research. This is true insofar as the relationship between the researcher and the participant in the research is unique and can never be completely replicated, although the same procedures and techniques may be followed and adopted. The research approach may be similar. Researchers must show their *audit trail* so that it is open to public scrutiny and subsequent researchers can follow it.

RESEARCH AIM

The aim of a research project is the researcher's intention to find out something about a *phenomenon* in a particular way in order to answer the *research question*. The aim of a qualitative study is generally fairly broad and uses terms such as 'explore, examine,' etc. A study might state the following for instance: 'The aim of this study is to gain insight into the experiences of patients in hospital.'

RESEARCH DESIGN

The research design is a plan of action for a research *proposal* in which researchers describe how they proceed and which strategies and *methods* they will adopt. Its components are: the collection and analysis of *data*, the intended development and extension of theory, and the process of establishing *validity* and *reliability* (trustworthiness and authenticity). In *qualitative research*, the design is flexible (Bogdan & Biklen, 1992); nevertheless, a clear design is necessary to make the study consistent and systematic within a flexible frame. Although researchers draw up an outline and boundaries, they develop and adjust the design during the process of the research, and they will decide on particular processes throughout the study. For instance, early assumptions might be wrong. During the course of the research, participants follow different directions from those envisaged initially. When this happens researchers might wish to modify their research design. (More detailed questions of design are described in the sections on specific approaches.)

RESEARCH QUESTION(S)

A research question is a **general question** about the *phenomenon* under study and what researchers wish to learn or understand about it. It is, of course, related to the problem that researchers want to examine and which the research aims to answer. It is formulated in general terms. Research questions are often developed at the start of a project but in qualitative research there is an ongoing process of formulating and modifying them and therefore the researcher should be able to adapt and be flexible. Maxwell (1996) suggests that questions that deal with the meaning of the phenomenon for the *participants* and its *context*, are more appropriate for *qualitative research* than questions that focus on causal explanations or on observed differences. The latter are better researched through quantitative methods. Maxwell (1992) gives three main types of *research questions*, as follows.

❏ **Descriptive questions** demand answers about behaviour or events in a setting or situation
❏ **Interpretive questions** ask about the *meaning* that situations or actions have for the participants and their feelings and intentions
❏ **Theoretical questions** are intended to provide reasons for actions or incidents in a particular situation

The research questions are quite different from the more specific questions asked in interviews: the former provide a framework for the understanding of a phenomenon whereas the interview questions are intended to produce the data for the answers to the research questions.

RESEARCH RELATIONSHIP

This is the relationship between the researcher and the other *participants* in the research. In qualitative research the relationship between the investigator and the participant differs from that in quantitative methodology. In the latter, researchers detach themselves from the participants in their inquiry who are seen as 'subjects' whose views can be examined from the outside. Quantitative researchers believe that this is more objective and produces better *data*. Qualitative researchers believe this detachment to be mechanistic; participants become passive 'subjects' and are seen as unequal. Qualitative researchers are not detached from the informants but become close to them and consider them as people. This is to some extent an outcome of the 'immersion' in the setting and 'prolonged engagement' with the participants.

The interaction between researcher and researched becomes an integral part of the research. The researcher approaches the participants as fully equal human beings. The relationship in much qualitative research is reciprocal and this allows the participant a position of **partnership** with the researcher (this emphasis on reciprocity is particularly strong in feminist research). Valuing others, adopting a **position of equality** towards the clients and empathising with them, while seeing them as human beings and not numbers, are principles inherent in qualitative research.

The researcher takes a **non-judgemental** stance towards the thoughts and words of the participants. Rapport and empathy are not only good qualities but also help in uncovering and producing rich data. The listener becomes the learner in this situation while the informant is the teacher. Rapport does not automatically imply an intimate relationship or deep friendship (Spradley, 1979), but it does lead to negotiation and sharing of ideas. It makes the research more interesting for the participants because they feel able to ask questions. Questions about the nature of the research project should be answered as honestly and openly as possible without creating bias in the study.

Hammersley & Atkinson (1995) point to the importance of **impression management** (a term used by Goffman (1969)), that is, the way people present themselves to others. They present through manner and demeanour as well as through outside appearance and clothing. Researchers might find making links easier if they dress appropriately for the situation. For instance, many nurse researchers adopt 'mufti' – non-uniform, ordinary clothing – when interviewing patients, in order to differentiate between their roles as researchers and those as professional carers and to avoid intimidation or formal situations. Teacher researchers would wear formal clothing when interviewing a head teacher whereas they would appear casually dressed at a school leisure centre. Through adopting an open and friendly manner, researchers relax the participants. Over time, the *research relationship* generates unofficial accounts from participants.

RESEARCH REPORT

The research report is the written document that researchers submit to others at the end of the research. It may take the form of a report for a commissioning or funding agency, a dissertation or thesis to be presented at an educational institution such as a university, or an article for peer review in an academic journal. Although conventions for writing up exist, they vary from one institution or agency to another. Qualitative writing may differ substantially from a quantitative report although commonalities exist. The main distinction lies in the flexibility writers have in writing up the qualitative report.

There is a difference between reports for practitioners in the professional setting, a report for a major funding body and a research dissertation or thesis. Employers and practitioners are most interested in the results and implications of the research for practice and less concerned with philosophical and theoretical issues while editors of academic journals see these as important. In a public report the participant's anonymity and confidentiality are protected.

The organisation of the report

Generally, writers organise their dissertation or thesis in the following sequence:

Title
Abstract
Acknowledgement and dedication
Table of contents
Introduction
    Background and justification of the study
    The aim of the research
    Initial *literature review* (or overview of the literature)
Methodology and *methods*
    Description and justification of methodology
        (including type of theoretical framework such as *symbolic interactionism*
        or *phenomenology*)
    The sample and the setting
    Specific procedures for data collection
    Data analysis

(contd)

Ethics
Findings/results and discussion
    (The findings and discussion are the most important elements of the final
      write-up and in consequence contain more words)
Conclusion and implications
    (Implications and/or recommendations are necessary for applied research
      in the professions, for instance)
References
Appendices

RESEARCH TOOL

In *qualitative research*, the researcher is the main research tool or instrument because researchers are intimately involved in the *context* and the setting. Their unique style and narration are an integral part of the study. Hence the **first person** 'I' is used in the description of the methodology or in the justification of the research in the introduction rather than 'the researcher' or 'the author', which sounds distant and uninvolved.

RIVAL EXPLANATION

A rival explanation is an alternative account of the events or phenomenon under study from that which the researcher has given. Qualitative researchers are aware that other explanations exist and must choose the strongest and most credible of several explanations (Miles & Huberman, 1994). This is only possible after intensive analysis, and therefore *premature closure* should be avoided.

S

SAMPLING

Qualitative sampling is generally **purposive** or purposeful. LeCompte & Preissle (1993) prefer the term **criterion-based sampling**, because qualitative researchers choose certain criteria in advance of their study on which the selection of a sample is based. In purposive sampling *generalisability* is less important than the collection of rich data and an understanding of the ideas of the people chosen for the sample. Patton (1990) lists 15 types of sampling in qualitative research.

Researchers choose a group or a number of individuals in whom they have an interest. These may be the members of a *culture* or a community who have knowledge of the setting or *phenomenon* under study. These *key informants* have had experience of an event or condition and are informed about the culture or topic area under investigation. In some cases a convenience sample can be justified. This means that researchers have convenient *access* to a number of *participants* and interview these for their study. Occasionally, snowball or chain-referral sampling is carried out: the informants recommend others who are able to give similar information because they have had similar experiences. For instance, a health professional might wish to interview people with a rare condition. These individuals might know others with the same condition whom they recommend for interviews. In interviews with people who wish to stay completely anonymous, even to the researcher, chain-referral sampling is useful.

Sampling decisions not only include people but can also involve sampling of events and concepts, time, processes and places (see *time sampling*). In purposive sampling researchers seek to gain as much knowledge as possible about the *context*, the person or other sampling units. This means that the sampling is not fixed in advance but is an ongoing process guided by emerging ideas.

The **sample size** in *qualitative research* is relatively small but consists of 'information-rich' cases (large samples are rarely selected). In-depth interviews and immersion in a culture make a large sample size unnecessary, particularly as qualitative researchers rarely seek to generalise. Generally the chosen sample includes between four and forty participants. For funded research Morse (1994) suggests a sample of about six in phenomenological studies because researchers search for the essence and richness of informants' experience, and a larger sample of around 30–50 for *grounded theory*. A small sample is sufficient when the researchers have chosen a homogeneous group or when they wish to investigate unusual or atypical phenomena. Indeed, in the latter case a sample of one might be sufficient. The sample size should be larger if it consists of a heterogeneous group of people. Maxwell (1996) adds that only when qualitative researchers aim for generalisability, might random sampling be used. This procedure can also be justified in projects with large numbers of volunteers so that researchers are seen to avoid preferential treatment in choosing the sample. The sample in qualitative research is rarely very large.

As qualitative researchers do not know the number of people in the sample before the research starts, the sample may change during the research in size and type. Sampling goes on until *saturation* has been achieved; that is, until no new information is generated and **informational redundancy** has occurred (Lincoln & Guba, 1985). According to Rubin & Rubin (1995), one of the main principles of sampling in qualitative research is completeness. Grounded theorists use **theoretical sampling**; this is sampling based on the developing *concepts* that appear important to the emerging *theory*. Sampling continues to *saturation*. (See *grounded theory*.)

Sandelowski (1995) recommends that researchers use their judgement about the numbers in the sample. Beginning qualitative researchers, she suggests, need larger sampling units than experienced researchers. She also reminds us that the sample does not consist merely of people but also of events and experiences. People are chosen mainly for their knowledge of an experience and condition or event about which they can speak to researchers.

SATURATION

This term is used in *grounded theory* in particular. Saturation occurs when further theoretical sampling does not uncover new ideas when researchers include additional participants. This happens when researchers are reasonably satisfied that they have exhaustively analysed the phenomenon under study, and when a full picture of the theoretical ideas emerges. The sampling has then reached completeness (Rubin & Rubin, 1995). This specific stage is called saturation point. (See **grounded theory**.)

SELF-DISCLOSURE

Self-disclosure in research is a revelation of experiences and feelings that are personal and private and have been hidden. Researchers must be sensitive in this situation and respect the rules of confidentiality unless the *participants* give their permission to uncover these feelings in the *research report*.

Self-disclosure is also an admission by researchers that they had similar experiences and perceptions to the participants. Sometimes this self-revelation originates in a genuine desire to share experiences, or even to be helpful; occasionally researchers take this path to generate deeper and more interesting responses. Feminists stress the importance of self-disclosure in their attempt to achieve equality between researcher and researched. Hammersley & Atkinson (1995) point to the occasional dangers of self-disclosure, particularly when the researcher's beliefs differ from those of the participants.

SENSITIZING CONCEPTS

Sensitizing concepts are ideas that guide the researcher towards particular events or behaviours in the setting. The term was used by Blumer (1954). These concepts provide foci for *observation* and *interviews*. Van den Hoonard (1997) describes sensitizing concepts as *constructs* which help guide researchers towards particular pathways for the research and are necessary for the development of an analytic framework. The concepts give insight into the social world and social processes (van den Hoonard demonstrates this by Goffman's concept of 'stigma' or Hochschild's term 'emotion work'). The use of sensitizing concepts is one of the traits which distinguishes qualitative from quantitative research.

Van den Hoonard claims that the 'discovery of grounded theory' (Glaser & Strauss, 1967) derives directly from Blumer's 'sensitizing concepts'. While qualitative researchers initially use inductive procedures, they do not enter the setting with 'tabula rasa', that is, their mind is not blank; they are already sensitive to the emerging concepts through experience and reading. They also arrive at sensitizing concepts through the ideas from the participants themselves. Sensitizing concepts are of obvious importance to qualitative research, particularly while theoretical sampling in *grounded theory* takes place. The term 'awareness context' used by Glaser & Strauss (1965), for instance, has become a 'sensitizing concept' in a number of nursing studies. While collecting and analysing their data, researchers trawl the literature related to the study and use ideas from reading as sensitizing devices. (See *literature review*.)

SERENDIPITY

Serendipity is an accidental lucky discovery which cannot be foreseen. Qualitative researchers sometimes find by chance an important idea, datum or sample unit that helps in the development of the research. These unanticipated findings often lead to unexpected directions. (According to the *Concise Oxford Dictionary*, 1995, the term 'serendipitous' was first used by Hugh Walpole in 1754 after the fairy tale 'The Three Princes of Serendip'.)

SETTING

The setting is the location where the research takes place. Researchers search for an appropriate setting. For *qualitative research*, they have to know the setting intimately, and for those who examine their own setting it is not difficult. Researchers generally describe in detail the settings in which the research takes place so that the reader can visualise it. Some settings are inappropriate and not feasible for the particular *research question*. In larger qualitative studies, it is useful to study more than one setting.

SOCIAL CONSTRUCTIONISM

Social constructionism, or constructivism, is a theoretical approach to social science which is based on the assumption that people construct their own social world. It focuses on their *meaning* and motives. Individuals are seen as active and competent human agents who build the social world in communication with each other, and there is doubt about the existence of objective knowledge. Many qualitative research approaches are founded on this belief-system which is well established in both sociology and psychology (Lincoln & Guba, 1990; Burr, 1995). Others maintain that radical *relativism* is an extreme position (Hammersley, 1992; Kelle & Laurie, 1995). Psychologists favour the term 'social constructionism' as constructivism could be mistaken for the direction in art called by the same name (Gergen, 1985). The term constructivism is popular in sociology where it is seen as less reductionist and limiting than social constructionism (although the latter term is also used).

Although many social scientists have worked within the framework of constructionism, the major development came from Berger & Luckmann's book *The Social Construction of Reality* (1967) although the term originated in

Schütz's work. Constructionists do not believe in a world 'out there' independent of human beings and a reification of the social world (see also *foundationalism*). As individuals and groups see the world differently, '**multiple realities**' – group and individual versions of reality – exist, and these are relative to *culture*, history and location. The constructions of human beings are not static but are changing continuously. Researchers who adopt this approach believe that the researcher and researched produce the findings of research together. Many constructionists adopt a relativist position to scientific knowledge (see *relativism*), seeing it, too, as a social construct. Others, although accepting this tenet, do not believe it to be merely a social construct (Richardson, 1996) but one that has some factual basis in empirical reality. The debate centres around the issue of discovery or creation of reality. W.J. Potter (1996) asserts that this problem can never be solved as the existence of an independent world or a socially created world cannot be empirically proven. Most social and indeed natural scientists believe in an independent external reality while they see the social world as constructed by human agents.

SPECIFICITY

Specificity exists when a specific situation or an individual case is examined, and when researchers do not seek generalisability. Much *qualitative research* has specificity.

SPONSORSHIP

The people who commission or fund a particular research project are its sponsors. Researchers must negotiate with the funding bodies or grant-giving agencies. Sometimes the sponsors determine the research topic; more usually it is developed jointly between researcher and sponsor. However, occasionally major funding bodies fund projects suggested by researchers, particularly when the research is seen as significant to achieve the aims of the sponsors or is for the benefit of their clients. In Britain, the National Health Service funds health research, and the Economic and Social Research Council (*ESRC*) funds economic and social research projects. The research report is generally presented in a way that fulfils the needs of the funding agency. Research carried out for a research degree at a university is not always sponsored. Most other types of research, however, are funded by outside bodies.

A number of problems arise through sponsorship. Some funding agencies try to direct or influence the research. As they are paying for it, they have, of course, the right to do so, especially as far as the *research question* is concerned. The problem arises when they also want to make decisions about methods and strategies for the research as they are not always knowledgeable about the best methods for a research question. This often happened in the past when a researcher chose a qualitative approach because most agencies were only familiar with quasi-experimental or survey methods. Qualitative approaches are, however, becoming more acceptable, and many fund-holding bodies have members with knowledge of qualitative research. The ESRC, for instance, funds good qualitative projects.

The funding of the project depends on the clarity of the research *proposal*, particularly its aims and objectives. In qualitative inquiry, objectives are not always stated because they often develop during the research process. The significance of the research and its justification are also important. Researchers take into account the type of grant-giving agency and its membership and functions, and write their proposals to fit in with the demands of the agency without losing their integrity.

STAKEHOLDER

The term 'stakeholder' is occasionally used in *qualitative research* instead of the term 'informant'. It is particularly popular in forms of *co-operative inquiry* and feminist approaches because the *participants* have a stake in the research and are equal partners with the researcher. The funding body is also sometimes called the stakeholder.

STORY

The story is the core of the qualitative *research report*, the essential content, or the *narrative*. Qualitative researchers tell a story which should be vivid and interesting as well as credible to the reader, and not merely entertaining but informative. This sometimes means writing and rewriting drafts until the *storyline* can be discerned clearly. There should be an accurate and systematic analysis of the *data* and a discussion of the results. The story contains the message with a set of ideas and beliefs. The events, the people and their words and actions are made explicit, so that readers can experience the situation as real in a similar way to the researcher and experience the world of the *participants*.

STORYLINE

The storyline is the *core category* in a *grounded theory* study that links all the categories and integrates the literature: in Strauss & Corbin's (1990: 116) words: 'the conceptualisation of the story'. Researchers identify and commit themselves to a *story* but should also be able to change it if the *data* demand this. The storyline is important for *grounded theory* and also for other types of *qualitative research*.

STORY TELLING

Participants give lengthy accounts and descriptions of their actions or feelings. Participants tell stories to the researcher in a *narrative* or a *life history*. These can be given verbally or in writing.

Qualitative researchers, too, are story tellers. Although the data collection and analysis are systematic and the *audit trail* is written in the form of a report, the findings and discussion should read like an interesting and lively story with a distinct *storyline*. It must be remembered though that the reader cannot always see the hard work which has gone into the development of a story, nor the complexities of strategy and procedure that produce it.

SUBJECTIVITY

Subjectivity here denotes the subjectivity of researchers (although qualitative inquiry also aims to identify and comprehend the subjective perspectives of the participants). In *qualitative research* subjectivity is usually seen as a potential resource. **Objectivity** is difficult to obtain due to the closeness of the relationship and the immersion in the setting, and because the qualitative researcher is the main research tool. The researchers' identities and experiences impinge on their work while they record what they hear, feel and see.

Much research deals with human beings, and this makes achieving objectivity more difficult. Instead of searching for explanation, prediction and control, the qualitative researcher seeks understanding of human thought and behaviour and its interpretation by the participants involved. This type of inquiry cannot be completely objective and neutral. The **prolonged immersion** in the setting and the close relationship with the participants make value neutrality and objectivity difficult.

Subjectivity sensitises researchers to the events and the people under investigation and may become a resource for the study. However, researchers must be reflexive and aware of their own assumptions while taking account of their own position (Olesen, 1994). Researchers might not recognise their subjectivity; it is difficult to be always conscious of one's own 'cultural baggage'. Researchers bring to the inquiry their own personalities, values and life experience and have to recognise and openly acknowledge their subjectivity.

The qualitative researcher recognises that social reality is constructed and depends on culture, time and place as well as on the individuals who observe the situation and interpret it. In qualitative research the subjective perspectives of participants and researcher become part of the study. The thoughts and values of the informants impinge on the research, but these are, of course, exactly that which the researchers want to explore. The investigators' own subjectivity becomes an analytic tool and is built into the research; they do not try to remove it. Using the self as a tool can help the researcher empathise and build relationships with the informants. Qualitative researchers must, however, attempt to disregard their own wishes to achieve a particular outcome. The concept of objectivity here does not mean a detached and neutral perspective but *reflexivity* about one's own values and an explicit description of one's culture, background and beliefs which might affect the research. All good researchers make sure that they carry out research without distorting what they see or hear. In this sense, qualitative researchers should be objective. They too should be open to 'alternative explanations'. A description by researchers of their subjectivity makes the research more objective (Banister *et al.*, 1994).

Reason & Heron (1995) use the term **critical subjectivity**. The subjective experience is a basis for knowledge, but this knowledge should not be accepted in a naïve way but be rooted in critical consciousness. Phenomenologists use *bracketing* which means that researchers explore their own assumptions and preconceptions in order to set them aside rather than concealing them. They are conscious of their own subjectivity and do not see it as a limitation or constraint. The researcher is self-critical and explicit.

The description of the methodological decisions made (the *audit trail*) means that readers and reviewers as well as other researchers can discover the subjective ideas of the investigator. The research is open to public scrutiny. Researchers try to be aware of their own assumptions and make them explicit so that the readers can judge the quality of the research for themselves.

To some writers on social research (for instance Lincoln & Guba (1985) and other constructivists), the debate about objectivity demonstrates that there is no such thing as a single social reality or truth, but that 'multiple realities' exist. Kvale (1995) claims that the concern of social scientists with objectivity may well reflect doubts about an objective social reality and act as an assurance that it exists. Barone (1992) insists that the debate about objectivity and subjectivity is now dead, and that there is always interaction between the objective world which exists independent of the observer and the subjective view of the observer who interprets it. (See *objectivity*.)

SYMBOLIC INTERACTIONISM

Symbolic interactionism, a term coined by Herbert Blumer (1900–1987) in 1937, is an approach in sociology which focuses on the interaction of human beings and the roles which they have. The model of the person in symbolic interactionism is active and creative rather than passive.

Symbolic interactionists see human behaviour as essentially social behaviour constituted of social acts. The essence of society lies in joint action. The best known of the symbolic interactionists is George Herbert Mead (1863–1931). Mead (1934) sees the self as a social rather than a psychological *phenomenon*. Individuals respond to others and grasp their *meanings* through forms of communication such as language, gestures and facial expressions. By interpreting and defining each others' language and actions, they choose from an infinite variety of social roles. Members of society affect the development of a person's social self by their expectations and influence. Initially, individuals model their roles on the important people in their lives, 'significant others'; they learn to act according to others' expectations, thereby shaping their own behaviour. Eventually, the individual is able to take on a number of social roles simultaneously and can organise the roles taken from the society, group or community, the 'generalised other'. Mead compares this to a team game, where members of a team anticipate the behaviour of other players and can therefore play their own roles.

Symbolic interactionists explain how individuals attempt to fit their lines of action to those of others (Blumer, 1971), take account of each others' acts, interpret them and reorganise their own behaviour. People share the attitudes and responses to particular situations with members of their group. Hence members of a *culture* or community analyse the language, appearance and gestures of others in the same setting and act in accordance with their interpretations. On these perceptions they base their justifications for conduct which can only be understood in *context*.

Symbolic interactionism is the basis of much social research, in particular qualitative inquiry. The strategies of participant *observation* and in-depth *interviews* have their origin in this theoretical perspective. Approaches to the analysis of qualitative data such as *grounded theory* and *analytic induction* are based on symbolic interactionism. *Ethnomethodology* and *conversation analysis* are related to this approach. Denzin (1989a) links symbolic interactionism to naturalistic, qualitative research methods by stating that researchers must enter the world of interactive human beings to understand them. By doing this, they see the situation from the perspective of the participants rather than their own. This perspective can be uncovered by interviews, observations and diaries. Qualitative methods suit the theoretical assumptions of symbolic interactionism. People can be observed in the process of their work and their negotiations with others.

T

TABLE OF CONTENTS

The table of contents is found at the beginning of a research report to show its contents and the page numbers of its sections. It is sectioned into chapter headings and subheadings with page numbers. Most reports have a table of contents before its main chapters begin. It cannot, of course, be finished before the whole project is complete and written.

TACIT KNOWLEDGE

Tacit knowledge is knowledge that the members of a *culture* share and take for granted but do not openly articulate to each other. Members base their behaviour and interpretations of the world on tacit knowledge. Ethnographers and other social researchers are concerned with 'uncovering' and making explicit this tacit knowledge in their research.

Polanyi (1983) also has an interest in the 'tacit dimension' of knowledge, but conceives it differently. He asserts that human beings have the capacity to know without being able to tell how this happens: 'we can know more than we tell' (p. 4). Polanyi believes that even explicit knowledge is tacitly understood and 'rooted in tacit knowledge'. Knowledge is achieved through tacit processes. The understanding of these helps researchers grasp the essence of a *phenomenon*. The tacit dimension guides them to underlying *meanings* in the human experience and assists in making inferences.

THEMATIC ANALYSIS

Thematic analysis is an analysis where the researcher identifies *themes* and patterns in *interviews* through listening to tapes and reading transcripts. Although the term is mainly associated with phenomenology, most qualitative approaches include some form of thematic analysis because researchers are searching for themes. It involves searching the *data* for related *categories* with similar *meaning*. These are then grouped together and **themes inferred** and generated from the data. Sometimes the themes are immediately obvious, but often the researchers must work hard to find them. The themes are then arranged for **thematic significance**.

Researchers engage in moving from the analysis back to the whole text and vice versa in order to develop new understanding and new questions. This allows comprehension of the participants' meanings, including inconsistencies and ambiguities.

THEME

A theme is a cluster of linked *categories* conveying similar *meanings* and forming a unit. Qualitative researchers often use the terms construct and theme interchangeably.

THEORETICAL SATURATION

Theoretical saturation in *qualitative research* is achieved through interaction between *data collection* and analysis. The term is used specifically in *grounded theory*. Saturation has taken place when no additional relevant data can be found and no new ideas for the development of theory arise. *Sampling* goes on until categories, their properties and dimensions as well as the links between the categories are well established. The theory will not be adequate unless this saturation has been achieved.

THEORETICAL SENSITIVITY

This means that the researcher is sensitive to the important issues in the data. The term was originally used by Glaser (1978) who believed that sensitivity assists the researchers in developing theories. Theoretical sensitivity derives from professional and personal experience. A thorough knowledge of the relevant literature and interaction with and immersion in the *data* also contribute to this awareness.

THEORY

Theory is a complex term that has more than one specific meaning. It is a grouping of related *concepts* and propositions with 'explanatory power'. Social theorists distinguish between types of *theory*, for instance grand theory, middle-range theory, substantive theory and formal theory; the latter two are developed in *grounded theory* and are of particular interest to qualitative researchers. **Substantive theory** is specific and refers to a substantive area of study whereas **formal theory** is developed at a conceptual and more general level (Strauss, 1987). The place of theory in qualitative research is unlike that in quantitative approaches; the relationship between theory and data is also different. Qualitative researchers, in particular those using grounded theory research, engage in theory building. A theory is generated from knowledge about specific instances and examples; that is, it is built on the information gained from the data. However, it must be stated that not all qualitative research has a developing theory (Morse & Field, 1996). *Phenomenology*, for instance, is concerned with the description of experiences and the essences of phenomena.

In many forms of *qualitative research*, theory is generated (as, for instance, in *grounded theory*) throughout the *data analysis*. Researchers then speak of 'emerging theory'. Sometimes researchers look for 'fit' between existing theories and the data collected, but the data are never forced into theory.

THICK DESCRIPTION

This term, coined by the philosopher Ryle (1949), was used by the anthropologist Geertz (1973) who applied it to *ethnography*. The detailed account of field experiences makes explicit the patterns of cultural and social relationships and puts them in *context*. It is a result of *observations* in the field. The notion of thick description is often misunderstood. It must be theoretical and analytical in that researchers concern themselves with the abstract and general patterns and traits of social life in a culture. This type of description aims to give readers a sense of the emotions, thoughts and perceptions that research participants experience. It deals not only with the meaning and interpretations of people in a culture but also with their intentions. Thick description builds up a clear picture of the individuals and groups in the context of their culture and the setting in which they live.

Thick description can be contrasted with **thin description**, which is a superficial account and does not explore the underlying meanings of cultural members. A study with thin description is not a good ethnography.

TIME SAMPLING

Time sampling means that the researcher visits a place or a person at different times of the day or week to gather *data* as the time of the *observation* or *interview* affects the nature of the data. For example, a nurse researcher might observe a ward setting in the morning or in the afternoon; and a teacher could observe a class when learners arrive and when they leave.

TIMELINE

The timeline gives the timetable for the planned work, and it is generally included in timetable format at the end of the *proposal*. When setting up their timetable, researchers should not forget to indicate that data collection and analysis proceed in parallel in qualitative research.

TITLE

The title of a study is the heading of the project, dissertation or thesis and presents an idea about the content. Occasionally it is given to researchers by funding bodies or stakeholders. The title should be concise but informative and reflect the aim of the research, but the aim does not need to be stated in detail in the title. It is initially a working title and may change when some of the research has been carried out. The *methodology* need not be included in the title. For instance, the title: 'The experience of people with epilepsy: a qualitative study', does not need the words 'a qualitative study'. Often researchers include other redundancies in the title such as 'A study of...', 'Aspects of...' or 'Inquiry into...', 'Analysis of...' or 'Investigation of...'. These are unnecessary and clumsy.

The title is the first and most immediate contact the reader has with the research and is therefore very important. The following are examples of short titles which give an indication of the studies' content: 'The pain career of people with chronic back pain' (Holloway *et al.*, 1996), 'When gender is not enough' (Riessman, 1987), and *Outsiders: Studies in the Sociology of Deviance* (Becker, 1963).

TITLE PAGE

The title page of a dissertation or thesis is the first page in the report. It contains the title, the name of the researcher, the date of the dissertation, and the name of the educational institution where the student was enrolled. There is generally a pro forma for the title page at most universities.

TOPIC SELECTION

The selection of the area to be studied depends on the researchers' interest and experience as well as on the relevance for the proposed readership. The topic should be suitable for *qualitative research*. Researchers also take into account the feasibility of the study, that is, whether they can investigate it in the time and locations available.

TRANSCRIPT

Transcripts are usually typed or hand-written passages made from tape recordings of *interviews* with *participants*, but also *fieldnotes* from observations and comments of the researcher. The face sheet of the transcripts should include the time, date and place of the interview as well as the pseudonym and code number of the participant. A brief description of the setting in which the interview takes place might be useful. The list of *participant* names and numbers should be stored away from the actual transcripts. It is also essential to indicate the type of transcript (for instance FN for fieldnotes, or IT for interview transcript). All pages must be numbered. **Wide margins** are important because coding and notes can be placed on the transcript. This should be larger on one side where the data can be coded and categorised. There is a space between the questions of the interviewer and those of the informant. It is important to make several copies of the transcript, one without comments or codes, and it should be put aside safely in case it needs to be re-coded or something happens to the copies.

Tapes are generally transcribed verbatim, including informants' errors of speech and repetitions as well as bridging phrases such as 'you know'. A full transcription of the tape would be most appropriate, although researchers may transcribe selectively (when transcribing their own tapes). Selective transcripts of sections of tape are permissible in later stages of the research process, though it is better to transcribe the whole tape. In textual analyses such as *conversation analysis*, transcriptions are essential. Transcribing a one-hour *interview* may take four hours or sometimes longer, depending on the skill of the transcriber or typist, the quality of the tape and the language and terms used. It is easier to analyse the data on a typed rather than hand-written transcript. An audio-machine with an on-off pedal is very useful for transcribing. Several **transcribing conventions** exist: they are most important for *conversation analysis* and for *discourse analysis*. Commonly, italics are used to stress words which the participant emphasised. Three full stops ... , indicate a pause, three spaced full stops, ... , show that lines or words have been left out. Two dashes with a question mark in the middle, /?/, indicate that the words or sentences in the tape could not be heard. Many researchers use their own system for transcribing tapes but a common **notation system** helps interviewers to remember these conventions.

Everything on the tape is of importance. Laughs or coughs should also be mentioned in the transcript, such as [laugh] or [slight cough], as they may indicate a feeling. Transcribing interviews gives the researcher an opportunity to get immersed in the *data*.

Transcripts contain the raw data from the participants but it should be realised that they have already undergone a process of transformation because gestures, mime or tone of voice cannot be duplicated in a transcript. O'Connell

& Kowal (1995: 105), however, stress that 'transcripts cannot take the place of the primary data base'.

TRIANGULATION

Triangulation is a process by which the same problem or phenomenon is investigated from different perspectives. It is sometimes believed that triangulation can improve *validity* and overcome the biases inherent in a single perspective. The *metaphor* triangulation stems originally from ancient Greek mathematics, and is now used in topographic surveying and navigation as a checking system where a point is 'fixed' or 'sighted' from different angles. In other words, to fix a point, observers sight the thing they want to locate from at least two different positions. The object is located at the point where the two lines intersect (Woolgar, 1988).

In research there are three main types of triangulation.

❏ between-methods (inter-method or across method) triangulation
❏ within-method (intra-method) triangulation
❏ investigator triangulation.

Researchers use **between-method triangulation** to confirm the findings generated through one particular method by another. **Within-method triangulation** adopts different strategies but stays within a single paradigm; for instance, participant observation and open-ended interviews are often used together in one qualitative study. Many qualitative researchers prefer within-method triangulation, because they claim that different methods have their origin in different world views and one researcher cannot have these views of the world at one and the same time (Leininger, 1992). Other researchers are more pragmatic.

Denzin (1989b) differentiates between four main types of triangulation, namely that of data, investigators, theories and methodologies. In **data triangulation**, researchers gain their data from different groups, locations and times. For instance, instead of collecting data from nurses in one community hospital, nurses in all the community hospitals in the area might be interviewed. Theory triangulation is the use of different theoretical perspectives in the study of one problem. **Investigator triangulation** means that more than one researcher is involved in the research. Becker *et al.* (1961) triangulated this way as several investigators were involved in their study of socialisation.

Data triangulation is different from **mixing methods**. In triangulation the researchers approach the same problem in different ways or from different angles. When they mix methods, they look at different problems in the same research study using different approaches. For instance, researchers might wish to follow up a few individuals from the sample of a survey population to explore their feelings about the factual issues that emerged in the survey. Researchers could use an exploratory study to identify issues for or refine the questionnaire.

TYPOLOGY

A typology is a classification scheme by which researchers group data, people or places into distinct and discrete types and label them. For this classification researchers seek to uncover dimensions or criteria by which these data, places and people differ. This system permits the researcher to divide, differentiate and understand differences between classes or groups. Researchers usually typologise on more than one dimension, but the classes or types into which they group people as well as events or settings must be meaningful. **Typologising** may mean oversimplification as it sometimes ignores complexities, particularly in the classification of people. Also, it is not the end stage of the research but researchers have to develop ideas about the dimensions and differences. For instance, nurse researchers might group patients into a typology of worried, calm, easy and 'difficult'; a teacher might talk about lazy students. Glaser (1978) differentiates between social scientists' typologies such as 'the high achiever' and lay typologies such as heroes and villains. Most social researchers and lay persons produce typologies when observing people.

V

VALIDITY

Validity is the scientific concept of the everyday notion of truth. All research must show that it has truth value. There are a variety of definitions of validity. The most common definition states that it is the extent to which an instrument measures what it is supposed to measure. In qualitative research it is the extent to which the findings of the study are true and accurate. Here validity is the extent to which the researcher's findings accurately reflect the purpose of the study and represent reality.

Validity is an important element that establishes the truth and authenticity of a piece of research, together with *reliability*. Most agree that in *qualitative research* understanding is more important than conventional notions of validity (Maxwell, 1992; Wolcott, 1995). Yonge & Stewin (1988) claim that the terms validity and reliability are misnomers in qualitative research. Nevertheless, qualitative researchers, too, have to establish the truth value of their research. It is perhaps more important in qualitative approaches because the concepts of validity and reliability are more problematic. Maxwell, however, does not see qualitative and quantitative perspectives on validity as incompatible.

On the issues of validity and reliability in qualitative research, two main strands of thought exist, although there is much discussion about these terms. Kvale (1989) and LeCompte & Preissle (1993) see the terms validity and reliability as justifiable in all research. Kirk & Miller (1986) and Maxwell (1996, 1992) also argue for the retention of these concepts in qualitative research, although they stress that qualitative researchers adopt different procedures to establish validity and reliability than researchers who use quantitative approaches. Internal validity is seen as the most important aspect of validity, and in qualitative research it has priority. The latter is seen as having high **internal validity:** researchers demonstrate that they present the reality of participants through a coherent storyline and excerpts from their interviews. Through the detailed description of the decision trail and their fieldnotes, they attempt to give evidence that they have portrayed the participants and the setting truthfully. Schofield (1993) suggests a coherent description of the situation under study consistent with the evidence which supports it. Internal validity is achieved when the researcher can demonstrate that there is evidence for the statements and descriptions made. The research is then open to public scrutiny.

External validity – the *generalisability* of the research – is more difficult to establish. Often, qualitative research is very specific to a particular location and place. Strauss & Corbin (1990) stress that theoretical concepts should have generalisability (and transferability). These concepts should be applicable to other, similar situations. This emphasises the vital importance of *thick description* so that the reader has the knowledge on which to base judgements. External validity is also enhanced when researchers choose a situation and setting which is typical of its kind (Schofield, 1993).

Guba (1981), Lincoln & Guba (1985), Guba & Lincoln (1989) and Erlandson *et al*. (1993) have long maintained that quality in qualitative research should be assessed differently from quantitative research. Others follow their ideas (Sandelowski, 1986; Koch, 1994, 1996). They provide alternative criteria because qualitative research differs inherently from quantitative inquiry, and adopt instead the notions of **trustworthiness** and authenticity. Trustworthiness (the qualitative researcher's alternative to validity) is the truth value of a piece of research. Qualitative research is trustworthy when it reflects the reality and the ideas of the participants. For Lincoln & Guba (1985) trustworthiness involves the following: credibility, transferability, dependability and confirmability.

Elements of trustworthiness

Credibility
Credibility corresponds to internal validity in quantitative research. It exists when the participants in a study recognise the truth of the findings in their own social context. This means that the researcher's findings are compatible with the perceptions of the people under study. It can be achieved through immersion in the setting (or 'prolonged engagement' and 'persistent observation'), meaning that researchers are involved intensely in the setting and with the participants over a considerable amount of time. *Triangulation* – the use of different methods or researchers and evidence from different sources of data – is another check on the truth value. A *member check* is a useful device: researchers verify their findings through feedback from the participants to whom they return with the findings and interpretations of their study. Finally Lincoln & Guba (1985) suggest *peer*

(contd)

debriefing. This means that researchers find out whether their colleagues arrive at similar interpretations when shown the data or the analysis.

Transferability

Transferability, the alternative term for external validity and generalisability, means that the findings in one context can be transferred to similar situations or participants. Lincoln & Guba (1985) also suggest that researchers use thick description and that they describe accurately and in detail the data in their context so that peers and readers have a clear picture of what goes on. Through purposeful sampling, too, rich and specific information is obtained.

Dependability

If a study is to be judged dependable (alternative term to reliable), it must be consistent and accurate. This can be demonstrated through an *audit trail* in which researchers provide detailed descriptions of the path of the research, so that readers can follow the decision-making process (it is also called decision trail by some researchers such as Sandelowski (1983) and Koch, 1994). Peers and readers are then able to carry out an ***inquiry audit*** in which they follow the path of the research.

Confirmability

The concept of confirmability (the equivalent of *objectivity*) means that the findings are the result of the research and not an outcome of the *biases* and *subjectivity* of the researcher. To achieve this, researchers have to uncover the decision trail for public judgement. Although qualitative researchers realise the futility of attempting to achieve objectivity, they must nevertheless be reflexive and show that the *data* can be traced back to their origins. Here, too, the audit trail, used to demonstrate dependability, should give the 'auditor' or the researcher's peer an opportunity to assess the findings of the study.

The other term used by Lincoln & Guba (1985) is authenticity. A study is authentic when the strategies used are appropriate for the true reporting of the participants' ideas. Authenticity consists of the following: fairness, ontological authenticity, educative authenticity, catalytic authenticity and tactical authenticity.

Components of authenticity

Fairness
Research must be fair to participants and gain their acceptance throughout the whole of the study. Continued informed consent must be obtained. The social *context* in which the *participants* work and live must also be taken into account.

Ontological authenticity
This means that participants gain an understanding of their human condition through the research.

Educative authenticity
The understanding that individuals gain should enhance the way in which they understand other people.

Catalytic authenticity
Decisions that are made by the participants which follow the research should be enhanced by the method of inquiry.

Tactical authenticity
After decisions are made, the actions of the participants should have an impact on their lives. The research should empower them.

It can be seen that these criteria are alternative and different from those of quantitative research. Nevertheless, it is important for qualitative research that its truth value be established.

VALUE NEUTRALITY

This concept means freedom from personal values. In the past, researchers and other social scientists were advised to be value neutral and not let their personal ideas influence their research. This value freedom is now seen as impossible. **Value commitment** is an adherence to a specific moral and value stance. For instance, feminist researchers are committed to the value of equality. Qualitative researchers have the responsibility to make their value commitment clear to the readers of the study and must avoid distortion by personal bias. (See *subjectivity*.)

VERSTEHEN

Verstehen (German for 'understanding'), according to Max Weber (1968), means understanding the point of view – the subjective meaning – of the other person. The origin of this idea lies in the writing of Dilthey (1833–1911), the German philosopher who initially developed the idea of **empathetic understanding**. The concept contains within it elements of interpretation. Verstehen, in Weber's view, distinguishes social from natural science. Researchers should be concerned with the interpretive understanding of the social actor's meaningful conduct. Meaning is found in the intentions and goals of the individual. This is the link to *qualitative research* where context of research and intent of participants are seen as important. The social observer interprets the meanings that people give to their behaviour.

Platt (1985) argues that Weber had no real association with qualitative research, and in particular participant observation as we know it today, partly because his work had not been translated at the time when qualitative research first became popular, partly because other theorists (such as Cooley or Mead) were better known at the time. One might argue though that Weber's ideas form links to qualitative research; they are now – though perhaps retrospectively – used and reviewed by qualitative researchers.

VIGNETTE

A vignette is an illustration or simulation of a typical event or phenomenon in the researcher's area of study. It is a brief description or an outline which demonstrates what is happening, and it is presented in story form. According to Miles & Huberman (1994: 83) a vignette 'is a concrete, focused story'. It is not an extended tale but a detailed abstraction of the event or phenomenon it describes. Researchers can introduce a topic through vignettes and ask questions about the area of research by presenting the vignettes to the participants. (Vignettes are frequently used in survey research. However, they can also assist qualitative researchers.)

References

Addison, R.B. (1992) Grounded hermeneutic research. In: *Doing Qualitative Research* (eds B.F. Crabtree & W.L. Miller), pp. 110–24, Sage, Thousand Oaks.

Agar, M. (1990) Exploring the excluded middle. *Journal of Contemporary Ethnography*, **19** (1) April. Special Issue: The Presentation of Ethnographic Research, 73–88.

Ashworth, P. (1993) Participant agreement in the justification of qualitative findings. *Journal of Phenomenological Psychology*, **24** (1), 3–16.

Atkinson, J.M. & Heritage, J. (eds) (1984) *Structures of Social Action: Studies in Conversation Analysis*. Cambridge University Press, Cambridge.

Atkinson, P. (1990) *The Ethnographic Imagination: Textual Constructions of Reality*. Routledge, London.

Atkinson, P. (1992) *Understanding Ethnographic Texts*. Sage, Newbury Park.

Atkinson, P. (1995) Some perils of paradigms. *Qualitative Health Research*, **5** (1), 117–24.

Baker, C., Wuest, J. & Stern, P.N. (1992) Method slurring: the grounded theory/phenomenology example. *Journal of Advanced Nursing*, **17**, 1355–60.

Banister, P., Bruman, E., Parker, I., Taylor, M. & Tindall, C. (1994) *Qualitative Methods in Psychology: A Research Guide*. Open University Press, Milton Keynes.

Barone, T.E. (1992) On the demise of subjectivity in educational inquiry. *Curriculum Inquiry*, **22** (1), 25–8.

Becker, H.S. (1963) *Outsiders: Studies in the Sociology of Deviance*. Free Press, New York.

Becker, H.S., Geer, B., Hughes, E. & Strauss, A.L. (1961) *Boys in White*. University of Chicago Press, New Brunswick.

Becker, P.H. (1993) Common pitfalls in grounded theory research. *Qualitative Health Research*, **3** (2), 254–60.

Benner, P. (ed.) (1994) *Interpretive Phenomenology: Embodiment, Caring and Ethics in Health and Illness*. Sage, Thousand Oaks.

Benner, P. (1994) The tradition and skill of interpretive phenomenology in studying health, illness and caring practices. In: *Interpretive Phenomenology: Embodiment, Caring and Ethics in Health and Illness* (ed. P. Benner), pp. 99–127. Sage, Thousand Oaks.

Berelson, B. (1952) *Content Analysis in Communication Research*. Free Press, Glencoe, Ill.

Berger, P. & Luckmann, T. (1967) *The Social Construction of Reality*. Allan Lane, London.

Blumer, H. (1954) What's wrong with social theory. *American Sociological Review*, **19**, 3–10.

Blumer, H. (1971) Sociological implications of the thoughts of G. H. Mead. In: *School and Society* (eds B.R. Cosin *et al.*), pp. 11–17. Open University Press, Milton Keynes.

Boas, F. (1928) *Anthropology and Modern Life*. Norton, New York.

Bogdan, R.C. & Biklen, S.K. (1992) *Qualitative Research for Education: An Introduction to Theory and Methods*, 2nd edn. Allyn & Bacon, Boston.

Bogdewic, S.P. (1992) Participant observation. In: *Doing Qualitative Research*. Research Methods in Primary Care (Vol. 3) (eds B.F. Crabtree & W.L. Miller), pp. 45–69. Sage, Newbury Park.

Bruner, J. (1987) Life as narrative. *Social Research*, **54** (1), 11–32.

Bryman, A. (1988) *Quantity and Quality in Social Research*. Unwin Hyman, London.

Burgess, R.G. (1984) *In the Field*. Allen & Unwin, London.

Burgess, R.G. (ed.) (1985) *Issues in Educational Research: Qualitative Methods*. Falmer, Lewes.

Burnard, P. (1992) Some problems in understanding other people: analysing talk in research, counselling and psychotherapy. *Nurse Education Today*, **12**, 130–36.

Burr, V. (1995) *An Introduction to Social Constructionism*. Routledge, London.

Carey, M.A. & Smith, M.W. (1994) Capturing the group effect in focus groups. *Qualitative Health Research*, **4** (1), 123–7.

Carr, W. & Kemmis, S. (1986) *Becoming Critical: Education, Knowledge and Action Research*. Falmer Press, London.

Chalmers, A.F. (1982) *What is this Thing called Science?* Open University Press, Milton Keynes.

Charmaz, K. (1995) Grounded theory. In: *Rethinking Methods in Psychology* (eds J.A. Smith, R. Harré & L. Van Langenhove), pp. 27–49. Sage, London.

Clarke, L. (1995) Nursing research: science, visions and telling stories. *Journal of Advanced Nursing*, **21**, 584–93.

Coffey, A. & Atkinson, P. (1996) *Making Sense of Qualitative Data: Complementary Research Strategies*. Sage, Thousand Oaks.

Cohen, M.Z. (1987) A historical overview of the phenomenologic movement. *Image: The Journal of Nursing Scholarship*, **19** (1), 31–4.

Colaizzi, P.F. (1978) Psychological research as the phenomenologist views it. In: *Existential Phenomenological Alternatives for Psychology* (eds R.S. Valle & M. King), pp. 48–71. Oxford University Press, New York.

Corbin, J. & Strauss, A. L. (1990) Grounded theory research: procedures, canons and evaluative criteria. *Qualitative Sociology*, **13** (1), 3–21.

Cormack, D.F.S. (1996) The critical incident technique. In: *The Research Process in Nursing* (ed. D.F.S. Cormack), 3rd edn, pp. 266–74, Blackwell Science, Oxford.

Corner, J. (1991) In search of more complete answers to questions: Quantitative versus qualitative methods, is there a way forward? *Journal of Advanced Nursing*, **16**, 718–27.

Corti, L., Foster, J. & Thompson, P. (1996) The need for a qualitative data archival policy. *Qualitative Health Research*, **6** (1), 135–9.

Couchman, W. & Dawson, J. (1995) *Nursing and Health-care Research*, 2nd edn. Scutari Press, London.

Crabtree, B.F. & Miller, W.L. (eds) (1992) *Doing Qualitative Research*. Sage, Thousand Oaks.

Cresswell, J.W. (1994) *Research Design: Qualitative and Quantitative Approaches*. Sage, Thousand Oaks.

Crotty, M. (1996) *Phenomenology and Nursing Research*. Churchill Livingstone, Melbourne.

Datta, L. (1994) Paradigm wars: A basis for peaceful coexistence and beyond. *New Directions for Program Evaluation*, **61**, 53–70.

Delamont, S. (1984) *Interaction in the Classroom*, 2nd edn. Methuen, London.

Delamont, S. (1992) *Fieldwork in Educational Settings: Methods, Pitfalls and Perspectives*. Falmer Press, London.

Delamont, S. & Atkinson, P.A. (1995) *Fighting Familiarity: Essays on Education and Ethnography*. Hampton Press, Cresskill, NJ.

Denny, T. (1978) Story telling and educational understanding. Paper presented at meeting of the International Reading Association, Houston, Texas. (ERIC Document Reproduction Service No. ED 170 314).

Denzin, N.K. (1989a) *Interpretive Interactionism*. Sage, Newbury Park.

Denzin, N.K. (1989b) *The Research Act: A Theoretical Introduction to Sociological Methods*, 3rd edn. Prentice-Hall, Englewood Cliffs, NJ.

Denzin, N.K. (1989c) *Interpretive Biography*. Sage, Newbury Park.

Denzin, N.K. & Lincoln, Y.S. (1994) Introduction: entering the field of qualitative research. In: *Handbook of Qualitative Research* (eds N.K. Denzin & Y.S. Lincoln), pp. 1–22. Sage, Thousand Oaks.

DePoy, E. & Gitlin, L.N. (1993) *Introduction to Research: Multiple Strategies for Health and Human Services*. Mosby, St Louis.

Deutscher, I. (1970) Words and deeds: social science and social policy. In: *Qualitative Methodology: Firsthand Involvement with the Social World* (ed. W.J. Filstead), pp. 27–51. Markham Publishing, Chicago.

Dey, I. (1993) *Qualitative Data Analysis*. Routledge, London.

Dickinson, H. & Erben, M. (1995) Bernstein and Ricoeur: Contours for the Social Understanding of Narratives and Selves. In: *Discourse and Reproduction* (eds P. Atkinson, B. Davies & S. Delamont), pp. 253–68. Hampton Press, Cresskill, NJ.

Duffy, M.E. (1985) Designing nursing research: The qualitative–quantitative debate. *Journal of Advanced Nursing*, **10**, 225–31.

Easthope, G. (1974) *A History of Social Research Methods*. Longman, London.

Erlandson, D.A., Harris, E.L., Skipper, B.L. & Allen, S.D. (1993) *Doing Naturalistic Research*. Sage, Newbury Park.

Fetterman, D.M. (1989) *Ethnography: Step by Step Sage*. Newbury Park.

Field, P.A. & Morse, J.M. (1985) *Nursing Research: The Application of Qualitative Approaches*. Croom Helm, London.

Fielding, N. (1981) *The National Front*. Routledge & Kegan Paul, London.

Fielding, N. & Lee, R. (eds) (1991) *Using Computers in Qualitative Research*. Sage, London.

Filstead, W.J. (ed.) (1970) *Qualitative Methodology: Firsthand Involvement with the Social World*. Markham Publishing, Chicago.

Finch, J. & Mason, J. (1990) Decision taking in the fieldwork process: Theoretical sampling and collaborative working. In: *Studies in Qualitative Methodology: Reflections on Field Experience* (ed. R.G. Burgess), pp. 25–50. JAI Press, Greenwich, CT, and, London.

Flanagan, J. (1954) The critical incident technique. *Psychological Bulletin*, **51**, 327–58.

Gadamer, H. (1960) *Truth and Method*. Sheed and Ward, London.

Garfinkel, H. (1967) *Studies in Ethnomethodology*. Prentice Hall, Englewood Cliffs.

Geertz, C. (1973) *The Interpretation of Cultures*. Basic Books, New York.

Geertz, C. (1976) From the native's point of view: On the nature of anthropological understanding. In: *Meaning in Anthropology* (eds K.H. Basso & H.A. Selby), pp. 221–37. University of New Mexico Press, Albuquerque.

Geertz, C. (1988) *Works and Lives: The Anthropologist as Author*. Polity Press, Cambridge.

Gergen, K.J. (1985) The social constructionist movement in modern psychology. *American Psychologist*, **40**, 266–75.

Gill, R. (1996) Discourse analysis: practical implementation. In: *Handbook of Qualitative Research Methods in Psychology and the Social Sciences* (ed. J.T.E. Richardson), pp. 141–56, BPS Books, Leicester.

Giorgi, A. (1975) An application of phenomenological method. In: *Duquesne Studies in Phenomenological Psychology* (eds A. Giorgi, C. Fischer & E. Murray), Vol. 2. Duquesne University Press, Pittsburgh, PA.

Giorgi, A. (1985) (ed.) *Phenomenology and Psychological Research*. Duquesne University Press, Pittsburgh, PA.

Giorgi, A., Fischer, W.F. & Von Eckartsberg, R. (1971) (eds) *Duquesne Studies in Phenomenological Psychology*, Vol. 1. Duquesne University Press, Pittsburgh, PA.

Glaser, B.G. (1978) *Theoretical Sensitivity*. Sociology Press, Mill Valley, CA.

Glaser, B.G. (1992) *Emergence versus Forcing: Basics of Grounded Theory Analysis*. Sociology Press, Mill Valley, CA.

Glaser, B.G. & Strauss, A.L. (1965) *Awareness of Dying*. Aldine, Chicago.

Glaser, B.G. & Strauss, A.L. (1967) *The Discovery of Grounded Theory*. Aldine, Chicago.

Glaser, B.G. & Strauss, A.L. (1968) *Time for Dying*. Aldine, Chicago.

Goffman, E. (1969) *The Presentation of Self in Everyday Life*. Penguin, Harmondsworth.

Gold, R. (1958) Roles in sociological field observation. *Social Forces*, **36**, 217–23.

Goodson, I.F. (1992) *Studying Teachers' Lives*. Routledge, London.

Greenbaum, T.L. (1988) *The Practical Handbook and Guide to Focus Group Research*. Lexington Books, D.C. Heath and Co, Lexington.

Guba, E. (1981) Assessing the trustworthiness of naturalistic inquiries. *Educational Communication and Technology Journal*, **29**, 75–92.

Guba, E. & Lincoln, Y. (1989) *Fourth Generation Evaluation*. Sage, Newbury Park.

Habermas, J. (1972) *Knowledge and Human Interests*. Heinemann, London (published in German, 1968).

Habermas, J. (1974) *Theory and Practice*. Heinemann, London (published in German, 1973).

Halpern, E.S. (1983) *Auditing naturalistic inquiries: the development and application of a model*. Unpublished doctoral dissertation, Indiana University (cited by Rodgers & Cowles, 1993, *op. cit.*).

Hammersley, M. (1983) *The Ethnography of Schooling*. Nafferton, Driffield.

Hammersley, M. (1990) *Reading Ethnographic Research: A Critical Guide*. Longman, London.

Hammersley, M. (1992) Some reflections about ethnography and validity. *Qualitative Studies in Education*, **5**, 195–203.

Hammersley, M. & Atkinson, P. (1983) *Ethnography: Principles in Practice*. Tavistock, London.

Hammersley, M. & Atkinson, P. (1995) *Ethnography: Principles in Practice*, 2nd edn. Tavistock, London.

Harding, S. (1987) Introduction. In: *Feminism and Methodology* (ed. S. Harding), pp. 1–14. Indiana Press, Bloomington.

Harré, R. & Secord, P.F. (1972) *The Explanation of Social Behaviour*. Blackwell, Oxford.

Harris, M. (1976) History and significance of the emic/etic distinction. *Annual Review of Anthropology*, **5**, 329–50.

Hayano, D.M. (1979) Auto-ethnography. *Human Organization*, **38**, 99–104.

Headland, T.N., Pike, K.L. & Harris, M. (eds) (1990) *Emics and Etics: The Insider/ Outsider Debate*. Sage, Newbury Park.

Heidegger, M. (1962) *Being and Time*. Harper & Row, New York (originally published in German in 1927; published in English in 1962).

Heritage, J. (1988) Explanations as accounts: a conversation analytic perspective. In: *Analysing Everyday Explanation: A Casebook of Methods* (ed. C. Antaki), pp. 127–44, Sage, London.

Heron, J. (1971) *Experience and Method*. University of Surrey, Guildford.

Heron, J. (1996) *Co-operative Inquiry: Research into the Human Condition*. Sage, London.

Hitchcock, G. & Hughes, D. (1995) *Research and the Teacher; A Qualitative Introduction to School-Based Research*, 2nd edn. Routledge, London

Hoffart, N. (1991) A member check procedure to enhance rigor in naturalistic research. *Western Journal of Nursing Research*, **13**, 522–34.

Holloway, I., Sofier, B. & Walker, J. (1996) The pain career of people with chronic back pain. Paper presented at the *Third International Interdisciplinary Qualitative Health Research Conference*, Bournemouth University, 30 Oct–1 Nov.

Holsti, O. (1969) *Content Analysis for the Social Sciences and Humanities*. Addison-Wesley, Reading, MA.

Hudelson, P.M. (1994) *Qualitative Research for Health Programmes*. Division of Mental Health, World Health Organisation, Geneva.

Husserl, E. (1931) Ideas: *General Introduction to Pure Phenomenology*. Allen Lane, London.

Hycner, R.H. (1985) Some guidelines for the phenomenological analysis of interview data. *Human Studies*, **8**, 279–303.

Ives, E.D. (1995) *The Tape-Recorded Interview: A Manual for Fieldworkers in Folklore and Oral History*, 2nd edn. The University of Tennessee Press, Knoxville, TN.

Janesick, V.A. (1994) The dance of qualitative research design. In: *Handbook of Qualitative Research* (eds N.K. Denzin & Y.S. Lincoln), pp. 209–19. Sage, Thousand Oaks.

Jary, D. & Jary, J. (1991) *Collins Dictionary of Sociology*. Harper Collins, Glasgow.

Kelle, U. & Laurie, H. (1995) Computer use in qualitative research and issues of validity. In: *Computer-Aided Qualitative Data Analysis: Theory, Methods and Practice* (ed. U. Kelle), pp. 19–28. Sage, London.

Kirk, J. & Miller, M.A. (1986) *Reliability and Validity in Qualitative Research*. Sage, Newbury Park.

Kitzinger, J. (1994) The methodology of Focus Groups: the importance of interaction between research participants. *Sociology of Health & Illness*, **16** (1), 102–21.

Koch, T. (1996) Expanding the Conception of Rigour in Qualitative Research. Presentation at the *Third International Interdisciplinary Qualitative Health Research Conference*, Bournemouth University, 30 October–1 November.

Koch, T. (1994) Establishing rigour in qualitative research: The decision trail. *Journal of Advanced Nursing*, **19**, 976–86.

Kools, S., McCarthy, M., Durham, R. & Robrecht, L. (1996) Dimensional analysis: broadening the conception of grounded theory. *Qualitative Health Research*, **6**, (3), 312–30.

Krippendorf, K. (1980) *Content Analysis: An introduction to its methodology*. Sage, Newbury Park [mainly a discussion of quantitative content analysis].

Krueger, R.A. (ed.) (1994) *Focus Groups: A Practical Guide for Applied Research*, 2nd edn. Sage, Thousand Oaks.

Kuhn, T.S. (1970) *The Structure of Scientific Revolutions*, 2nd edn. University of Chicago Press, Chicago.

Kvale, S. (1989) *Issues of Validity in Qualitative Research*. Studentlitteratur, Lund.

Kvale, S. (1995) The social construction of validity. *Qualitative Inquiry*, **1**(1), 19–40.

LeCompte, M.D. & Preissle, J. with Tesch, R. (1993) *Ethnography and Qualitative Design in Educational Research*, 2nd edn. Academic Press, Chicago.

Leininger, M. (ed.) (1985) *Qualitative Research Methods in Nursing*. Grune & Stratton, New York.

Leininger, M. (1992) Current issues, problems, and trends to advance qualitative paradigmatic research methods for the future. *Qualitative Health Research*, **2** (4), 392–415.

Leudar, I. & Antaki, C. (1988) Completion and dynamics in explanation seeking. In: *Analysing Everyday Explanation: A Casebook of Methods* (ed. C. Antaki) pp. 145–55. Sage, London.

Lewin, K. (1946) Action research and minority problems. In: *Resolving Social Conflicts: Selected Papers on Group Dynamics by Kurt Lewin* (ed. G.W. Lewin). Harper and Brothers, New York.

Lewins, A. (1996) The CAQDAS networking project: multilevel support for the qualitative research community. *Qualitative Health Research*, **6** (2), 298–303.

Lincoln, Y.S. & Guba, E.G. (1985) *Naturalistic Inquiry*. Sage, Beverly Hills.

Lincoln, Y.S. & Guba, E.G. (1990) *The Paradigm Dialogue*. Sage, Newbury Park.

Lindemann, E.C. (1924) *Social Discovery*. Republic, New York.

Lindesmith, A.R. (1947) *Opiate Addiction*. Principia, Bloomington.

Locke, L., Spirduso, W.W. & Silverman, S.J. (1993) *Proposals that Work: a Guide for Planning Dissertations and Grant Proposals*, 3rd edn. Sage, Newbury Park.

Lofland, J. & Lofland, L. (1995) *Analysing Social Settings*, 3rd edn. Wadsworth, Belmont, CA.

McHoul, A. & Grace, W. (1995) *A Foucault Primer: Discourse, Power and the Subject*. UCL Press, London. First published in 1993 by Melbourne University Press.

Malinowski, B. (1922) *Argonauts of the Western Pacific: An Account of Native Enterprise and Adventure in the Archipelagoes of Melanesian New Guinea*. Dutton, New York.

Mangabeira, W.C. (ed.) (1996) Qualitative sociology and computer programs: advent and diffusion of CAQDAS. *Current Sociology*, **44** (3).

Manning, P. (1982) Analytic induction. In: *Qualitative Methods*, Vol. 2, *Handbook of Social Science Methods* (eds R. Smith & P.K. Manning), pp. 273–303. Ballinger, Cambridge, Mass.

Marshall, C. & Rossman, G.R. (1995) *Designing Qualitative Research*, 2nd edn. Sage, Thousand Oaks.

Marton, F. (1986) Phenomenography: a research approach to investigating different understandings of reality. *Journal of Thought*, **21**, 28–49.

Marton, F. (1981) Phenomenography: describing conceptions of the world around us. *Instructional Science*, **10**, 177–200.

Mason, J. (1996) *Qualitative Researching*. Sage, London.

Maxwell, J.A. (1992) Understanding and validity in qualitative research. *Harvard Educational Review*, **62**, 279–300.

Maxwell, J.A. (1996) *Qualitative Research Design: An Interactive Approach*. Sage, Thousand Oaks.

May, R.B., Masson, M.E.J. & Hunter, M.A. (1990) *Application of Statistics in Behavioural Research*. Harper & Row, New York.

Mays, M. & Pope, C. (Eds) (1996) *Qualitative Research in Health Care*. BMJ Publishing Group, London.

Mead, G.H. (1934) *Mind, Self and Society*. University of Chicago Press, Chicago.

Mead, M. (1935) *Sex and Temperament in Three Primitive Societies*. Morrow, New York.

Melia, K.M. (1987) *Learning and Working*. Tavistock, London.

Melia, K.M. (1996) Rediscovering Glaser. *Qualitative Health Research*, **6** (3), 368–78.

Merleau-Ponty, M. (1962) *Phenomenology of Perception*. Humanities Press, New York.

Merriam, S.J. (1988) *Case Study Research in Education*. Jossey Bass, San Francisco.

Miles, M.B. & Huberman, A.M. (1994) *Qualitative Data Analysis*, 2nd edn. Sage, Thousand Oaks.

Millett, K. (1969) *Sexual Politics*. Abacus, London.

Minichiello, V., Aroni, R., Timewell, E. & Alexander, L. (1990) *In-depth Interviewing: Researching People*. Longman Cheshire, Melbourne.

Mitchell, J. (1971) *Women's Estate*. Penguin, Harmondsworth.

Morgan, D.L. (1988) *Focus Groups as Qualitative Research*. Sage, Newbury Park. (There will be a 1997 edition).

Morgan, D.L. & Krueger, R.A. (1993) When to use Focus Groups and why. In: *Successful Focus Groups: Advancing the State of the Art* (ed. D.L. Morgan), pp. 3–19. Sage, Newbury Park.

Morse, J.M. (ed.) (1991a) *Qualitative Nursing Research: A Contemporary Dialogue*. Sage, Newbury Park.

Morse, J.M. (1991b) Subjects, respondents, informants and participants. *Qualitative Health Research*, **1**, 403–6.

Morse, J.M. (1994) Designing funded qualitative research. In: *Handbook of Qualitative Research* (eds N.K. Denzin & Y.S. Lincoln), pp. 220–235. Sage, Thousand Oaks.

Morse, J.M. & Field, P.A. (1996) *Nursing Research: The Application of Qualitative Approaches*, 2nd edn. Chapman & Hall, London.

Moustakas, C. (1990) *Heuristic Research*. Sage, Newbury Park.

Moustakas, C. (1994) *Phenomenological Research Methods*. Sage, Thousand Oaks.

Nicolson, P. (1991) Qualitative psychology: Report prepared for the Scientific Affairs Board of the British Psychological Society. Leicester, UK, as quoted in J.T.E. Richardson (1996) *Handbook of Qualitative Research Methods in Psychology and the Social Sciences*. BPS Books, Leicester.

Novak, J.D. & Gowin, D.B. (1984) *Learning How to Learn*. Cambridge University Press, Cambridge.

Oakley, A. (1972) *Sex, Gender and Society*. Temple Smith, London.

O'Connell, D.C. & Kowal, S. (1995) Basic principles of transcription. In: *Rethinking Methods in Psychology* (eds J. A. Smith, R. Harré & L. Van Langenhove), pp. 93–105. Sage, London.

Oiler Boyd, C. (1993) Phenomenology: the method. In: *Nursing Research: A Qualitative Perspective*, 2nd edn (eds P.L. Munhall & C. Oiler Boyd), pp. 99–132. National League for Nursing Press, New York.

Olesen, V. (1994) Feminism and models of qualitative research. In: *Handbook of*

Qualitative Research (eds N.K. Denzin & Y.S. Lincoln), pp. 158–74. Sage, Thousand Oaks.

Park, R. & Burgess, E. (1925) *The City*. University of Chicago Press, Chicago.

Patton, M.Q. (1990) *Qualitative Evaluation and Research Methods*, 2nd edn. Sage, Newbury Park.

Payne, G.C.F. & Cuff, E.C. (1982) *Doing Teaching*. Batsford, London.

Phillips, D.C. (1993) Subjectivity and objectivity: An objective inquiry. In: *Educational Research: Current Issues* (ed. M. Hammersley), pp. 57–72. Paul Chapman, London.

Pike, K.L. (1954) *Language in Relation to a Unified Theory of the Structure of Human Behaviour*. Summer Institute of Linguistics, Glendale, CA (and further editions of this book).

Platt, J. (1983) The development of the participant observation method in sociology: origin, myth and history. *Journal of the History of the Behavioral Sciences*, **19**, 379–93.

Platt, J. (1985) Weber's Verstehen and the history of qualitative research: the missing link. *British Journal of Sociology*, **36** (3), 448–66.

Polanyi, M. (1983) *The Tacit Dimension*. Peter Smith, Gloucester, MA.

Popper, K. (1959) *The Logic of Scientific Discovery*. Routledge & Kegan Paul, London.

Potter, J. (1996a) *Representing Reality: Discourse, Rhetoric and Social Construction*. Sage, London.

Potter, J. (1996b) Discourse analysis and constructionist approaches: theoretical background. In: *Handbook of Qualitative Research Methods in Psychology and the Social Sciences* (ed. J.T.E. Richardson), pp. 125–40. BPS Books, Leicester.

Potter, J. & Wetherell, M. (1987) *Discourse and Social Psychology: Beyond Attitudes and Behaviour*. Sage, London.

Potter, W.J. (1996) *An Analysis of Thinking and Research about Qualitative Methods*. Lawrence Erlbaum Associates, Mahwah, NJ.

Psathas, G. (1995) *Conversation Analysis: The Study-of-Talk-in-Interaction*. Sage, Thousand Oaks.

Reason, P. (ed.) (1994) *Participation in Human Inquiry*. Sage, London.

Reason, P. & Heron, J. (1995) Cooperative inquiry. In: *Rethinking Methods in Psychology* (eds J.A. Smith., R. Harré & L. Van Langenhove), pp. 122–42. Sage, London.

Reason, P. & Rowan, J. (1981) (eds) *Human Inquiry: A Sourcebook of New Paradigm Research*. Wiley, Chichester.

Reichardt, C.S. & Rallis, S.F. (1994) Qualitative and quantitative inquiries are not incompatible: A call for a new partnership. *New Directions for Program Evaluation*, **61**, 85–91.

Reinharz, S. (1993) Empty explanations for empty wombs: an illustration of a secondary analysis of qualitative data. In: *Qualitative Voices in Educational Research* (ed. Michael Schratz), pp. 157–78. Falmer Press, London.

Richardson, J.T.E. (ed.) (1996) *Handbook of Qualitative Research Methods for Psychology and the Social Sciences*. British Psychological Society, Leicester.

Ricoeur, P. (1984) *Time and Narrative, Vol. 1*. Chicago University Press, Chicago.

Ricoeur, P. (1985) *Time and Narrative, Vol. 2*. Chicago University Press, Chicago.

Riessman, C. (1987) When gender is not enough: Women interviewing women. *Gender and Society*, **1** (2), 172–207.

Riessman, C.K. (1993) *Narrative Analysis*. Sage, Newbury Park.

Robrecht, L. (1995) Grounded theory: evolving methods. *Qualitative Health Research*, **5** (2), 169–77.

Robson, C. (1993) *Real World Research*. Blackwell, Oxford.

Rodgers, B.L. & Cowles, K.V. (1993) The qualitative research audit trail. *Research in Nursing and Health*, **16**, 219–26.

Rubin, H.R. & Rubin, I.S. (1995) *Qualitative Interviewing*. Sage, Thousand Oaks.

Ryle, G. (1949) *The Concept of Mind*. Hutchinson, London.

Sandelowski, M. (1986) The problem of rigor in qualitative research. *Advances in Nursing Science*, **8**, 27–37.

Sandelowski, M. (1993) Rigor or rigor mortis: The problem of rigor in qualitative research revisited. *Advances in Nursing Science*, **16**, 1–8.

Sandelowski, M. (1994) The use of quotes in qualitative research. *Research in Nursing and Health*, **17**, 479–83.

Sandelowski, M. (1995) Sample size in qualitative research. *Research in Nursing and Health*, **18**, 179–83.

Sanger, J. (1996) *The Compleat Observer? A Field Research Guide to Observation*. Falmer Press, London.

Sarantakos, S. (1994) *Social Research*. Macmillan, London.

Sartre, J. (1965) *Being and Nothingness*. Citadel Press, New York. (Originally published in French, 1943.)

Schatzman, L. (1991) Dimensional analysis: notes on an alternative approach to the rounding of theory in qualitative research. In: *Social Organisation and Social Process: Essays in Honor of Anselm Strauss* (ed. D.R. Maines), pp. 303–14. Aldine de Gruyter, New York.

Schatzman, L. & Strauss, A.L. (1973) *Field Research: Strategies for a Natural Sociology*. Prentice Hall, Englewood Cliffs.

Schofield, J.W. (1993) Increasing the generalizability of qualitative research. In: *Educational Research: Current Issues* (ed. M. Hammersley), pp. 91–113. Paul Chapman, London.

Schütz, A. (1967) *The Phenomenology of the Social World*. Heinemann, London (originally published in German, 1932).

Schwandt, T. & Halpern, E.S. (1988) *Linking Auditing and Metaevaluation. Enhancing Quality in Applied Research*. Sage, Newbury Park.

Scott, B.S. & Lyman, S.N. (1972) Accounts. In: *Symbolic Interaction* (eds J.G. Manis & B.N. Meltzer), pp. 404–31. Allyn & Bacon, Boston.

Scott, J. (1990) *A Matter of Record: Documentary Sources in Social Research*. Polity Press, Cambridge.

Seidman, I.E. (1991) *Interviewing as Qualitative Research*. Teachers College, Columbia University, New York.

Shaffir, W.B. & Stebbins, R.A. (eds) (1991) *Experiencing Fieldwork*. Sage, Newbury Park.

Shelton-Reed, J. (1997) Narrative in sociological writing. Sociology Seminar at the University of Surrey, 30 January.

Sieber, J.E. (1992) *Planning Ethically Responsible Research*. Sage, London.

Silverman, D. (1993) *Interpreting Qualitative Data*. Sage, London.

Smith, J.A., Harré, R. & Van Langenhove, L. (1995) *Rethinking Methods in Psychology*. Sage, London.

Smith, J.K. (1983) Quantitative versus qualitative research: an attempt to clarify the issue. *Educational Researcher*, **12** (3), 6–13.

Smith, P. (1992) *The Emotional Labour of Nursing*. Macmillan Education, London.

Spiegelberg, H. (1960) *The Phenomenological Movement: A Historical Introduction* (Vols 1&2), 2nd edn. Nijhoff, The Hague.

Spradley, J.P. (1970) *You Owe Yourself a Drunk: An Ethnography of Urban Nomads*. Little, Brown & Co, Boston.

Spradley, J.P. (1979) *The Ethnographic Interview*. Harcourt Brace Jovanovich/College Publishers, Fort Worth.

Spradley J.P. (1980) *Participant Observation*. Harcourt Brace Jovanovich/College Publishers, Fort Worth.

Springer, E. T. (1996) *Action Research: A Handbook for Practitioners*. Sage, Thousand Oaks.

Stake, R.E. (1995) *The Art of Case Study Research*. Sage, Thousand Oaks.

Stanley, L. & Wise, S. (1993) *Breaking Out Again*. Routledge, London.

Stern, P.N. (1994) Eroding grounded theory. In: *Critical Issues in Qualitative Research Methods* (ed. J.M. Morse), pp. 212–23. Sage, Thousand Oaks.

Stewart, D.W. & Shamdasani, P.N. (1990) *Focus Groups, Theory and Practice*. Sage, Newbury Park.

Stockwell, F. (1984) *The Unpopular Patient*. Croom Helm, London.

Strauss, A.L. (1987) *Qualitative Analysis for Social Scientists*. Cambridge University Press, New York.

Strauss, A. & Corbin, J. (1990) *Basics of Qualitative Research: Grounded Theory Procedures and Techniques*. Sage, Newbury Park.

Strauss, A. & Corbin, J. (1994) Grounded theory methodology: an overview. In: *The Handbook of Qualitative Research* (eds N.K. Denzin & Y. Lincoln), pp. 173–285. Sage, Thousand Oaks.

Strauss, A.L., Schatzman, L., Bucher, R., Ehrlich, D. & Sabshin, M. (1964) *Psychiatric Ideologies and Institutions*. Collier Macmillan, London.

Streubert, H.J. & Carpenter, D.R. (1995) *Qualitative Research in Nursing: Advancing the Human Imperative*. J.B. Lippincott Co, Philadelphia, PA.

Tesch, R. (1990) *Qualitative Research: Analysis Types and Software Tools*. Falmer Press, London.

Tesch, R. (1991) Software for Qualitative Researchers. In: *Using Computers in Qualitative Research* (eds N.G. Fielding & R.M. Lee), pp. 16–37. Sage, London,

Thomas, J. (1993) *Doing Critical Ethnography*. Sage, Newbury Park.

Thomas, W.I. & Znaniecki, F. (1927) *The Polish Peasant in Europe and America* (2 vols). Alfred Knopf, New York.

Thompson, N. (1995) *Theory and Practice in Health and Social Care*. Open University Press, Milton Keynes.

Timmerman, G.M. (1996) The art of advertising for research subjects. *Nursing Research*, **45** (6), 339, 344.

Turner, R. (ed.) (1974) *Ethnomethodology*. Penguin Books, Harmondsworth.

Usher, R. & Bryant, I. (1989) *Adult Education as Theory, Practice and Research: The Captive Triangle*. Routledge, London.

Vallé, R.S. & King, M. (eds) (1978) *Existential Phenomenological Alternatives for Psychology*. Oxford University Press, New York.

van den Hoonaard, W.C. (1997) *Working with Sensitizing Concepts*. Sage, Thousand Oaks.

van Dijk, T.A. (ed.) (1985) *Discourse and Communication: New Approaches to the Analysis of Mass Media Discourse and Communication*. Walter de Gruyter, Berlin.

van Maanen, J. (1988) *Tales of the Field: On Writing Ethnography*. University of Chicago Press, Chicago.

van Manen, M. (1984) Practising phenomenological writing. *Phenomenology and Pedagogy*, **2** (1), 36–69.

van Manen, M. (1990) *Researching Lived Experience: Human Science for an Action Sensitive Pedagogy*. State University of New York Press, New York.

Watson, G. & Seiler, R.M. (eds) (1992) *Text in Context: Contributions to Ethnomethodology*. Sage, Newbury Park.

Webb, C. (1984) Feminist methodology in nursing research. *Journal of Advanced Nursing*, **9**, 249–56.

Webb, C. (1992) The use of the first person in academic writing: objectivity, language and gatekeeping. *Journal of Advanced Nursing*, **17**, 747–52.

Weber, M. (1968) *Economy and Society: An Outline of Interpretive Sociology*. Bedminster Press, New York (this is a translation, the original was written in 1922 as *Wirtschaft und Gesellschaft*).

Weiss, R.S. (1994) *Learning from Strangers: The Art and Method of Qualitative Interview Studies*. The Free Press, New York.

Werner, O. & Schoepfle, G.M. (1987) *Systematic Fieldwork: Vol. 1, Foundations of Ethnography and Interviewing*. Sage, Newbury Park.

Werner, O. & Schoepfle, G.M. (1987) *Systematic Fieldwork: Vol. 2, Ethnography Analysis and Data Management*. Sage, Newbury Park.

Westkott, M. (1990) Feminist criticism of the social sciences. In: *Feminist Research Methods. Exemplary Readings in the Social Sciences* (ed. J.M. Nielsen), pp. 58–68. Westview Press, London.

Whyte, W.F. (1943) *Street Corner Society: The Social Structure of an Italian Slum*. University of Chicago Press, Chicago.

Wilde, V. (1992) Controversial hypotheses on the relationship between researcher and informant in qualitative research. *Journal of Advanced Nursing*, **17**, 234–42.

Williams, M. & May, T. (1996) *Introduction to the Philosophy of Social Research*. UCL Press, London.

Wolcott, H.F. (1994) *Transforming Qualitative Data: Description, Analysis, and Interpretation*. Sage, Thousand Oaks.

Wolcott, H.F. (1995) *The Art of Fieldwork*. Altamira Press, Walnut Creek, CA.

Woolgar, S. (1988) *Science: The Very Idea*. Ellis Harwood, Chichester.

Woolsey, L.K. (1986) The critical incident technique: an innovative qualitative method of research. *Canadian Journal of Counselling*, **20** (4), 242–54.

Woods, P. (1979) *The Divided School*. Routledge & Kegan Paul, London.

Yin, R.K. (1993) *Applications of Case Study Research*. Sage, Newbury Park.

Yonge, O. & Stewin, L. (1988) Reliability and validity: misnomers for qualitative research. *Canadian Journal of Nursing Research*, **20** (2), 61–7.

Books for Qualitative Researchers

This is not a comprehensive list of books on qualitative research, methodology and procedures, nor does it include all early classic texts in this field. It is, I hope, reasonably extensive and up to date.

Introductory texts

Bailey, C.A. (1996) *A Guide to Field Research*. Pine Forge Press, Thousand Oaks.
Glesne, C. & Peshkin, A. (1992) *Becoming Qualitative Researchers: An Introduction*. Longman, New York.
Maykut, P. & Morehouse, R. (1994) *Beginning Qualitative Research: A Philosophic and Practical Guide*. Falmer Press, London.

General Texts
(These include texts on sociological and psychological qualitative research.)

Banister, P., Bruman, E., Parker, I., Taylor, M. & Tindall, C. (1994) *Qualitative Methods in Psychology: A Research Guide*. Open University Press, Milton Keynes.
Berg, D. (1995) *Qualitative Research Methods for the Social Sciences*. 3rd edn. Allyn & Bacon, Boston.
Bryman, A. (1988) *Quantity and Quality in Social Research*. Unwin Hyman, London.
Bryman, A. & Burgess, R.G. (1994) *Analysing Qualitative Data*. Routledge, London.
Coffey, A. & Atkinson, P. (1996) *Making Sense of Qualitative Data: Complementary Research Strategies*. Sage, Thousand Oaks.
Cresswell, J.W. (1994) *Research Design: Qualitative and Quantitative Approaches*. Sage, Thousand Oaks.
Denzin, N.K. & Lincoln, Y.S. (eds.) (1994) *Handbook of Qualitative Research*. Sage, Thousand Oaks.
Fielding, N.G. & Fielding, J.L. (1986) *Linking Data*. Sage, Beverly Hills.
Gubrium, J. (1988) *Analyzing Field Reality*. Sage, Beverley Hills.

Hammersley, M. & Atkinson, P. (1995) *Ethnography: Principles in Practice*, 2nd edn. Tavistock, London.

Hitchcock, G. & Hughes, D. (1995) *Research and the Teacher; A Qualitative Introduction to School-Based Research*, 2nd edn. Routledge, London.

Lincoln, Y.S. & Guba, E.G. (1985) *Naturalistic Inquiry*. Sage, Beverly Hills.

Lofland, J. & Lofland, L. (1995) *Analysing Social Settings*, 3rd edn. Wadsworth, Belmont.

Marshall, C. & Rossman, G.R. (1995) *Designing Qualitative Research*, 2nd edn. Sage, Thousand Oaks.

Mason, J. (1996) *Qualitative Researching*. Sage, London.

Maxwell, J.A. (1996) *Qualitative Research Design: An Interactive Approach*. Sage, Thousand Oaks.

Miller, G. & Dingwall, R. (eds) *Context and Method in Qualitative Research*. Sage, London.

Miles, M.B. & Huberman, A.M. (1994) *Qualitative Data Analysis*, 2nd edn. Sage, Thousand Oaks.

Patton, M.Q. (1987) *Qualitative Evaluation Research Methods*. Sage, Newbury Park.

Patton, M.Q. (1990) *Qualitative Evaluation and Research Methods*, 2nd edn. Sage, Newbury Park.

Potter, W.J. (1996) *An Analysis of Thinking and Research about Qualitative Methods*. Lawrence Erlbaum Associates, Mahwah, NJ.

Richardson, J.T.E. (ed.) (1996) *Handbook of Qualitative Research Methods for Psychology and the Social Sciences*. British Psychological Society, Leicester.

Schwandt, T.A. (1997) *Qualitative Inquiry: A Dictionary of Terms*. Sage, Thousand Oaks.

Silverman, D. (1985) *Qualitative Methodology and Sociology: Describing the Social World*. Gower, Aldershot.

Silverman, D. (1993) *Interpreting Qualitative Data*. Sage, London.

Silverman, D. (ed.) (1997) *Qualitative Research: Theory, Method and Practice*. Sage, Thousand Oaks.

Smith, J.A., Harré, R. & Van Langenhove, L. (1995) *Rethinking Methods in Psychology*. Sage, London. (This book does not merely describe qualitative approaches.)

Taylor, S.J. & Bogdan, R.C. (1984) *Introduction to Qualitative Research and Methods: The Search for Meaning*. Wiley, New York.

van Zuuren, E.J., Wertz, E.J. & Mook, B. (1987) *Advances in Qualitative Psychology: Themes and Variations*. Swets & Zeitlinger, Lisse, Holland.

Wolcott, H.F. (1994) *Transforming Qualitative Data: Description, Analysis, and Interpretation*. Sage, Thousand Oaks.

Practical help and guidance

Meloy, J.M. (1994) *Writing the Qualitative Dissertation: Understanding by Doing*. Lawrence Erlbaum Associates, Hillsdale, NJ.

Riley, J. (1990) *Getting the Most from Your Data: A Handbook of Practical Ideas on How to Analyse Your Data*. Technical and Educational Services, Bristol.

Wolcott, H.F. (1990) *Writing up qualitative research*. Sage, Newbury Park.

Fieldwork

Atkinson, P.A. (1991) *Field and Text*. Sage, Beverly Hills.
Burgess, R.G. (1984a) *In the Field*. Allen & Unwin, London.
Burgess, R.G. (1984b) *Strategies of Educational Research*. Falmer Press, London.
Burgess, R.G. (1985a) *Field Methods in the Study of Education*. Falmer Press, London.
Delamont, S. (1992) *Fieldwork in Educational Settings: Methods, Pitfalls and Perspectives*. Falmer Press, London.
Sanjek, R. (ed.) (1990) *Fieldnotes: The Makings of Anthropology*. Cornell University Press, Ithaca, NY.
van Maanen, J. (1988) *Tales of the Field: On Writing Ethnography*. University of Chicago Press, Chicago.
Whyte, W.F. (1984) *Learning from the Field*. Sage, Beverly Hills.
Wolcott, H.F. (1995) *The Art of Fieldwork*. Altamira Press, Walnut Creek, CA.

Data collection, sources and analysis

Focus groups
Carey, M.A. (ed.) (1995) Issues and applications of focus groups. *Special Issue: Qualitative Health Research*, **5** (4).
Greenbaum, T.L. (1988) *The Practical Handbook and Guide to Focus Group Research*. Lexington Books, D.C. Heath and Co, Lexington.
Krueger, R.A. (1988) *Focus Groups: A Practical Guide for Applied Research*. Sage, Newbury Park.
Krueger, R.A. (ed.) (1994) *Focus Groups: A Practical Guide for Applied Research*, 2nd edn. Sage, Thousand Oaks.
Merton, R.K. & King, R. (1990) *The Focused Interview: A Manual of Problems and Procedures*, 2nd edn. Free Press, New York.
Morgan, D.L. (1988) *Focus Groups as Qualitative Research*. Sage, Newbury Park.
Morgan, D.L. (ed.) (1993) *Successful Focus Groups: Advancing the State of the Art*. Sage, Newbury Park.
Stewart, D.W. & Shamdasani, P.N. (1990) *Focus Groups, Theory and Practice*. Sage, Newbury Park.

Interviewing
Chirban, J.T. (1996) *Interviewing in Depth. The Interactive–Relational Approach*. Sage, Thousand Oaks.
Holstein, J.A. & Gubrium, J.F. (1995) *The Active Interview*. Sage, Thousand Oaks.
Kvale, S. (1996) *InterViews: An Introduction to Qualitative Research Interviewing*. Sage, Thousand Oaks.

McCracken, G. (1988) *The Long Interview*. Sage, Newbury Park.

Minichiello, V., Aroni, R., Timewell, E. & Alexander, L. (1990) *In-depth Interviewing: Researching People*. Longman Cheshire, Melbourne.

Rubin, H.R. & Rubin, I.S. (1995) *Qualitative Interviewing*. Sage, Thousand Oaks.

Seidman, I.E. (1991) *Interviewing as Qualitative Research*. Teachers College, Columbia University, New York.

Spradley, J.P. (1979) *The Ethnographic Interview*, Harcourt Brace Jovanovich/College Publishers, Fort Worth, TX.

Weiss, R.S. (1994) *Learning from Strangers: The Art and Method of Qualitative Interview Studies*. Free Press, New York.

Narrative/life history

Cortazzi, M. (1993) *Narrative Analysis*. Falmer Press, London.

Denzin, N.K. (1989) *Interpretive Biography*. Sage, Newbury Park.

Hatch, J.A. & Wisniewski, R. (eds) (1995) *Life History and Narrative*. Falmer Press, London.

Josellson, R. & Lieblich, A. (1993) *The Narrative Study of Lives*. Sage, Newbury Park.

Mitchell, W.J. (ed.) (1991) *On Narrative*. University of Chicago Press, Chicago.

Plummer, K. (1983) *Documents of Life*. Allen & Unwin, London.

Riessman, C.K. (1993) *Narrative Analysis*. Sage, Newbury Park.

Rosenwald, G. & Ochburg, R. (eds) (1992) *Storied Lives*. Yale University Press, New Haven, CT.

Sarbin, T.R. (ed.) (1986) *Narrative Psychology: The Storied Nature of Human Conduct*. Praeger, New York.

Witherell, C. & Noddings, N. (eds) (1991) *The Stories Lives Tell: Narrative and Dialogue in Education*. Teachers College Press, Columbia University, NY.

Observation

Jorgenson, D.L. (1989) *Participant Observation*. Sage, Newbury Park.

Sanger, J. (1996) *The Compleat Observer? A Field Research Guide to Observation*. Falmer Press, London.

Spradley, J.P. (1980) *Participant Observation*. Harcourt Brace Jovanovich, Fort Worth, TX.

Theory and philosophy

Blaikie, N. (1993) *Approaches to Social Enquiry*. Polity Press, Cambridge.

Eisner, E.W. & Peshkin, A. (eds) (1990) *Qualitative Inquiry in Education; The Continuing Debate*. Teachers College Press, Columbia University, New York.

Flinders, D.J. & Mills, G.E. (eds) (1993) *Theory and Concepts in Qualitative Research; Perspectives from the Field*. Teachers College Press, Columbia University, New York.

Guba, E.G. (ed.) (1992) *The Paradigm Dialog*. Sage, Newbury Park.
Hammersley, M. (1995) *The Politics of Social Research*. Sage, London.
Hughes, J. (1990) *The Philosophy of Social Research*. Longman, London.
Layder, D. (1993) *New Strategies in Social Research*. Polity Press, Cambridge.
Silverman, D. (1985) *Qualitative Methodology and Sociology*. Gower, Aldershot.
Williams, M. & May, T. (1996) *Introduction to the Philosophy of Social Research*. UCL Press, London.

Texts for different methods and strategies

Action research and collaborative research

Fals-Borda, O. & Rahman, M.A. (eds) (1991) *Action and Knowledge: Breaking the Monopoly with Participative Action Research*. Intermediate Technology/Apex, New York.
Hart, E. & Bond, M. (1995) *Action Research for Health and Social Care*. Open University Press, Buckingham.
Heron, J. (1996) *Co-operative Inquiry: Research into the Human Condition*. Sage, London.
Reason, P. (ed.) (1988) *Human Inquiry in Action: Developments in New Paradigm Research*. Sage, London.
Reason, P. (ed.) (1994) *Participation in Human Inquiry*. Sage, Thousand Oaks.
Reason, P. & Rowan, J. (eds) (1981) *Human Inquiry: A Sourcebook for New Paradigm Research*. John Wiley, Chichester.
Springer, E.T. (1996) *Action Research: A Handbook for Practitioners*. Sage, Thousand Oaks.

Case study

Hamel, J. with Dufour, S. & Fortin, D. (1993) *Case Study Methods*. Sage, Newbury Park.
Merriam, S.J. (1988) *Case Study Research in Education*. Jossey Bass, San Francisco.
Stake, R.E. (1995) *The Art of Case Study Research*. Sage, Thousand Oaks.
Yin, R.K. (1993) *Applications of Case Study Research*. Sage, Newbury Park.
Yin, R.K. (1994) *Case Study Research*, 2nd edn. Sage, Thousand Oaks. (Books by Yin focus mainly on quantitative research, but mention qualitative approaches.)

Ethnography

Agar, M. (1986) *Speaking of Ethnography*. Sage, Newbury Park.
Agar, M. (1990) Exploring the excluded middle. *Journal of Contemporary Ethnography*, **19** (1), April Special Issue: The Presentation of Ethnographic Research, 73–88.
Agar, M. (1980) *The Professional Stranger: An Informal Introduction to Ethnography*. Sage, Newbury Park.
Atkinson, P. (1992) *Understanding Ethnographic Texts*. Sage, Newbury Park.

Denzin, N.K. (1997) *Interpretive Ethnography: Ethnographic Practices for the 21st Century*. Sage, Thousand Oaks.
Fetterman, D.M. (1989) *Ethnography: Step by Step*. Sage, Newbury Park.
Hammersley, M. (1990) *Reading Ethnographic Research*. Longman, London.
Hammersley, M. & Atkinson, P. (1995) *Ethnography: Principles in Practice*, 2nd edn. Tavistock, London.
LeCompte, M.D. & Preissle, J. with Tesch, R. (1993) *Ethnography and Qualitative Design in Educational Research*, 2nd edn. Academic Press, Chicago.
Spradley, J.P. (1979) *The Ethnographic Interview*. Harcourt Brace Jovanovich/College Publishers, Fort Worth, TX.
Thomas, J. (1993) *Doing Critical Ethnography*. Sage, Newbury Park.
van Maanen, J. (1988) *Tales of the Field: On Writing Ethnography*. University of Chicago Press, Chicago.
Werner, O. & Schoepfle, G.M. (1987) *Systematic Fieldwork: Vol. 1, Foundations of Ethnography and Interviewing*. Sage, Newbury Park.
Werner, O. & Schoepfle, G.M. (1987) *Systematic Fieldwork: Vol. 2, Ethnography Analysis and Data Management*. Sage, Newbury Park.
Wolcott, H.F. (1994) *Transforming Qualitative Data: Description, Analysis, and Interpretation*. Sage, Thousand Oaks.

Conversation analysis

Atkinson, J.M. & Heritage, J. (eds) (1984) *Structures of Social Action: Studies in Conversation Analysis*. Cambridge University Press, Cambridge.
Button, G. & Lee, J.R.E. (eds) (1987) *Talk and Social Organisation*. Multilingual Matters Ltd, Clevedon.
Nofsinger, R.E. (1991) *Everyday Conversation*. Sage, Newbury Park.
Psathas, G. (1995) *Conversation Analysis: The Study-of-Talk-in-Interaction*. Sage, Thousand Oaks.
Turner, R. (ed.) (1974) *Ethnomethodology*. Penguin Books, Harmondsworth.
Watson, G. & Seiler, R.M. (eds) (1992) *Text in Context: Contributions to Ethnomethodology*. Sage, Newbury Park.

Discourse analysis

Antaki, C. (ed.) (1988) *Analysing Everyday Explanation: A Casebook of Methods*. Sage, London.
Burman, E. & Parker, I. (eds) (1993) *Discourse Analytic Research: Readings and Repertoires of Texts in Action*. Routledge, London.
Burr, V. (1995) *An Introduction to Social Constructionism*. Routledge, London.
Edwards, D. (1996) *Discourse and Cognition*. Sage, London.
Edwards, J.A. & Lampert, M.D. (eds) (1993) *Talking Data: Transcription and Coding in Discourse Research*. Lawrence Erlbaum, Hillsdale, NJ.
Nunan, D. (1993) *Discourse Analysis*. Penguin, London.

Parker, I. (1992) *Discourse Dynamics: Critical Analysis for Social and Individual Psychology*. Routledge, London.

Potter, J. (1996) *Representing Reality: Discourse, Rhetoric and Social Construction*. Sage, London.

Feminist and anti-sexist research

Bowles, G. & Duelli Klein, R. (eds) (1983) *Theories of Women's Studies*. Routledge & Kegan Paul, London.

Eichler, M. (1988) *Nonsexist Research Methods: A Practical Guide*. Routledge, London.

Fonow, M.M. & Cook, J.A. (eds) (1991) *Beyond Methodology: Feminist Scholarship as Lived Research*. Bloomington, Indiana University Press.

Gilligan, C. (1982) *In a Different Voice*. Harvard University Press, Cambridge, MA.

Harding, S. (ed.) (1987) *Feminism and Methodology*. Indiana Press, Bloomington.

Lennon, K. & Whitford, M. (eds) (1994) *Knowing the Difference: Feminist Perspectives in Epistemology*. Routledge, London.

Nielsen, J.M. (ed.) (1990) *Feminist Research Methods. Exemplary Readings in the Social Sciences*. London, Westview Press.

Reinharz, S. (1992) *Feminist Methods in Social Research*. Oxford University Press, New York.

Stanley, L. & Wise, S. (1983) *Breaking Out: Feminist Consciousness and Feminist Research*. Routledge & Kegan Paul, London.

Stanley, L. & Wise, S. (1993) *Breaking Out Again*. Routledge, London.

Grounded theory

Glaser, B. G. (1978) *Theoretical Sensitivity*. Sociology Press, Mill Valley.

Glaser, B.G. (1992) *Basics of Grounded Theory Analysis*. Sociology Press, Mill Valley.

Glaser, B.G. & Strauss, A.L. (1967) *The Discovery of Grounded Theory*. Aldine Publishing, Chicago.

Schatzman, L. & Strauss, A.L. (1973) *Field Research: Strategies for a Natural Sociology*. Prentice Hall, Englewood Cliffs.

Strauss, A.L. (1987) *Qualitative Analysis for Social Scientists*. Cambridge University Press, New York.

Strauss, A. & Corbin, J. (1990) *Basics of Qualitative Research: Grounded Theory Procedures and Techniques*. Sage, Newbury Park.

Strauss, A.L. & Corbin, J. (eds) (1997) *Grounded Theory in Practice*. Sage, Thousand Oaks.

Wiener, C.L. & Wysmans, W.M. (eds) (1990) *Grounded Theory in Medical Research*. Swets & Zeitlinger, Amsterdam.

Phenomenology

Benner, P. (ed.) (1994) *Interpretive Phenomenology: Embodiment, Caring and Ethics in Health and Illness*. Sage, Thousand Oaks.

Crotty, M. (1996) *Phenomenology and Nursing Research*. Churchill Livingstone, Melbourne.

Karlsson, G. (1993) *Psychological Qualitative Research from a Phenomenological Perspective*. Department of Psychology, University of Stockholm, Stockholm.

Moustakas, C. (1994) *Phenomenological Research Methods*. Sage, Thousand Oaks.

van Manen, M. (1990) *Researching Lived Experience: Human Science for an Action Sensitive Pedagogy*. State University of New York Press, New York.

Qualitative evaluation research

Fink, A. (1993) *Evaluation Fundamentals: Guiding Health Programs, Research and Policy*. Sage, Newbury Park.

Guba, E. & Lincoln, Y. (1989) *Fourth Generation Evaluation*. Sage, Newbury Park.

Patton, M.Q. (1987) *Qualitative Evaluation Research Methods*. Sage, Newbury Park.

Worthen, B. & Saunders, J. (1987) *Educational Evaluation: Alternative Approaches and Practical Guidelines*. Longman, London.

Texts for different disciplines

Education

Bogdan, R.C. & Biklen, S.K. (1992) *Qualitative Research for Education: An Introduction to Theory and Methods*, 2nd edn. Allyn & Bacon, Boston.

Eisner, E.W. & Peshkin, A. (eds) (1990) *Qualitative Inquiry in Education: The Continuing Debate*. Teachers College Press, Columbia University, New York.

Hammersley, M. (ed.) (1983) *The Ethnography of Schooling: Methodological Issues*. Nafferton Books, Driffield.

Hitchcock, G. & Hughes, D. (1995) *Research and the Teacher: A Qualitative Introduction to School-based Research*, 2nd edn. Routledge, London.

LeCompte, M., Millroy, W.L. & Preissle, J. (eds) (1992) *Handbook of Qualitative Research in Education*. Academic Press, San Diego.

LeCompte, M.D. & Preissle, J. with Tesch, R. (1993) *Ethnography and Qualitative Design in Educational Research*, 2nd edn. Academic Press, Chicago.

Salisbury, J. & Delamont, S. (1995) *Qualitative Studies in Education*. Avebury Press, Aldershot.

Schratz, M. (ed.) (1993) *Qualitative Voices in Educational Research*. Falmer Press, London.

Spindler, G. (ed.) (1987) *Doing the Ethnography of Schooling*. Holt, Rinehart & Winston, New York.

Spindler, G. (ed.) (1987) *Interpretive Ethnography of Education: At Home and Abroad*. Lawrence Erlbaum Associates, London.

Sherman, R.R. & Webb, R. B. (eds) (1988) *Qualitative Research in Education: Focus and Methods*. Falmer Press, Philadelphia, PA.

van Manen, M. (1990) *Researching Lived Experience: Human Science for an Action Sensitive Pedagogy*. State Unversity of New York Press, New York.

Health care, medical and nursing research

Benner, P. (ed.) (1994) *Interpretive Phenomenology: Embodiment, Caring and Ethics in Health and Illness*. Sage, Thousand Oaks.

Bloor, M. & Taraborelli, P. (eds) (1994) *Qualitative Studies in Health and Medicine*. Avebury, Aldershot.

Chenitz, W.C. & Swanson, J.M. (eds.) (1986) *From Practice to Grounded Theory: Qualitative Research in Nursing*. Addison Wesley, Menlo Park.

Crabtree, B.F. & Miller, W.L. (eds) (1992) *Doing Qualitative Research*. Sage, Thousand Oaks.

Crotty, M. (1996) *Phenomenology and Nursing Research*. Churchill Livingstone, Melbourne.

Holloway, I. & Wheeler, S. (1996) *Qualitative Research for Nurses*. Blackwell Science, Oxford.

Hudelson, P.M. (1994) *Qualitative Research for Health Programmes*. Division of Mental Health, World Health Organization, Geneva.

Leininger, M. (ed.) (1985) *Qualitative Research Methods in Nursing*. Grune & Stratton, New York.

Mays, M. & Pope, C. (eds) (1996) *Qualitative Research in Health Care*. BMJ Publishing Group, London.

Morse, J.M. (ed.) (1991) *Qualitative Nursing Research: A Contemporary Dialogue*, revised edn. Sage, Newbury Park.

Morse, J.M. (ed.) (1992) *Qualitative Health Research*. Sage, Newbury Park.

Morse, J.M. (ed.) (1994) *Critical Issues in Qualitative Research*. Sage, Thousand Oaks.

Morse, J.M. & Field, P.A. (1996) *Nursing Research: The Application of Qualitative Approaches*, 2nd edn. Chapman & Hall, London.

Munhall, P.L. & Oiler Boyd, C. (eds) (1993) *Nursing Research: A Qualitative Perspective*, 2nd edn. National League for Nursing Press, New York.

Parse, R., Coyne, A. & Smith, M. (1985) *Nursing Research: Qualitative Methods*. Brady Communications, Bowie, MD.

Streubert, H.J. & Carpenter, D.R. (1995) *Qualitative Research in Nursing: Advancing the Human Imperative*. J.B. Lippincott Co, Philadelphia, PA.

Wiener, C.L. & Wysmans, W.M. (eds) (1990) *Grounded Theory in Medical Research*, Swets & Zeitlinger, Amsterdam.

Social work

Ferguson, P.M., Ferguson, D.L. & Taylor, S.J. (eds) (1992) *Interpreting Disability: A Qualitative Reader*. Teachers College Press, Columbia University, NY.

Martin, R. (1995) *Oral History in Social Work*. Sage, Thousand Oaks.

Riessman, C.K. (ed.) (1994) *Qualitative Studies in Social Work Research*. Sage, Thousand Oaks.

Sherman, E. & Reid, W.J. (eds) (1994) *Qualitative Research in Social Work*. Columbia University Press, New York and London.

Additional areas for qualitative research

Alasuntaari, P. (1995) *Researching Culture: Qualitative Method and Cultural Studies*. Sage, London.

Altheide, D.L. (1996) *Qualitative Media Analysis*. Sage, Thousand Oaks.

Gilgun, J.F., Daly, K. & Handel, G. (eds) (1992) *Qualitative Methods in Family Research*. Sage, Newbury Park.

Jensen, K.B. & Jankowski, W. (eds) (1995) *A Handbook of Qualitative Methodologies for Mass Communication Research*. Routledge, London.

Lindlof, T.R. (1995) *Qualitative Communication Research Methods*. Sage, Thousand Oaks.

Potter, W.J. (1996) *An Analysis of Thinking and Research about Qualitative Methods*. Lawrence Erlbaum Associates, Mahwah, NJ (media research).

Computers in qualitative research

Burgess, R.G. (ed.) (1995) *Studies in Qualitative Methodology: Computing and Qualitative Research*. JAI Press, Greenwich, CT, and London.

Dey, I. (1993) *Qualitative Data Analysis*. Routledge, London.

Fielding, N.G. & Lee, R.M. (eds) (1991) *Using Computers in Qualitative Research*. Sage, London.

Kelle, U. (ed.) (1995) *Computer-Aided Qualitative Data Analysis: Theory, Methods and Practice*. Sage, London.

Mangabeira, W.C. (ed.) (1996) Qualitative sociology and computer programs: advent and diffusion of CAQDAS. *Current Sociology*, **44** (3).

Pfaffenberger, B. (1988) *Microcomputer Applications in Qualitative Research*. Sage, Beverly Hills.

Tesch, R. (1990) *Qualitative Research: Analysis Types and Software Tools*. Falmer Press, London.

Weaver, A. & Atkinson, P. (1994) *Microcomputing and Qualitative Data Analysis*. Avebury, Aldershot.

Weitzman, E.A. & Miles, M.B. (1994) *Computer Aided Qualitative Data Analysis: A Review of Selected Software*. Center for Policy Research, New York.

There is also the Qualitative Research Method Series (Sage University Papers). Some of the texts in this series are given in the booklist above.